THE PLEASURES OF LOVE

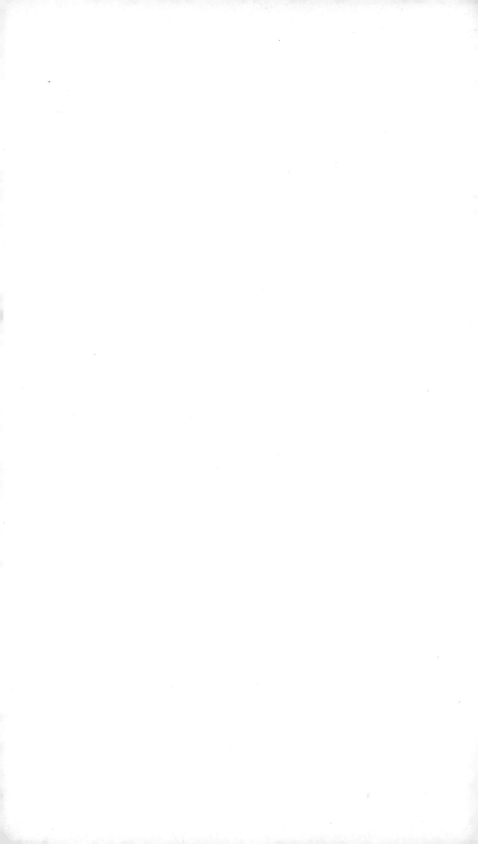

THE PLEASURES OF LOVE

The ultimate guide to sexual fulfilment for you and your partner.

Pierre and Marie Habert

foulsham
LONDON • NEW YORK • TORONTO • SYDNEY

foulsham
The Publishing House, Bennetts Close
Cippenham, Berkshire SL1 5AP, England.

Neither the editors of W. Foulsham & Co. Limited nor the authors or the publisher take responsibility for any possible consequences from any treatment, procedure, test, exercise, action or application of medication or preparation by any person reading or following the information in this book.

ISBN 0-572-02212-3

This English language edition copyright © 1997 W. Foulsham & Co. Ltd. Originally published by © Editions Solar with the design by Antoine Dumond and the photographs by l'Agence Vloo.

All rights reserved. The Copyright Act prohibits (subject to certain very limited exceptions) the making of copies of any copyright work or of a substantial part of such a work, including the making of copies by photocopying or similar process. Written permission to make a copy or copies must therefore normally be obtained from the publisher in advance. It is advisable also to consult the publisher if in any doubt as to the legality of any copying which is to be undertaken.

Translation by Julian Worthington
Typeset in Great Britain by Typesetting Solutions, Slough, Berks.
Text printed in Great Britain by St. Edmundsbury Press, Bury St. Edmunds, Suffolk.
Colour illustrations printed in Great Britain by Cambus Litho, East Kilbride.

CONTENTS

1 A MAN, A WOMAN: THE ENCOUNTER, THE DESIRE

- Love: the Happiness and the Tears 11
  Taking the rough with the smooth 12
  Expressing love in letters 13

- The Sensual Wealth of Your Body 16
  Discovering your femininity 16
  Discovering your male virility 25
  Test your erotic sensibility 29
  Pleasure on one's own 30

- Body Language 32
  Aids to seduction 34
  Getting rid of complexes 36
  Flirting: one step towards adult love 37

- Pleasure Comes from the Whole Body 39
  Kissing according to the Kama Sutra 41
  A turning-point in life 44
  Some testimonies 47

2 THE KNOW-HOW OF LOVE

- The Prelude: Body Talk 51
  Some testimonies 54

- The Sensual Message: Relaxation and Arousal 56

- The Most Intimate Love-making 58
  Fellatio 59

Cunnilingus	60
In what positions should one practise oral sex?	60
An intimate secret	60
Some testimonies	61
• **The Absolute Pleasure**	62
Orgasm ... dying of pleasure	62
What happens in the woman's body from foreplay to orgasm	65
What happens in the man's body from foreplay to orgasm	67
How to say it	70
• **Sexual Intercourse**	71
A little, a lot, passionately ... not at all	71
• **Pregnancy and Love**	74
The pregnant woman's reactions to sexual stimulation	77
Sex after childbirth	78

3 THE SOURCES OF EXCITEMENT

• **Fantasies: Your Secret Garden**	81
Andrea and the men in chains	83
Hugh and the fluffy toys	84
Richard and the air-hostesses	85
Nadine and the young blonde	86
• **Fetishism: Objects of Desire**	88
Some testimonies	90
• **Voyeurism: A Certain Look**	91
Some testimonies	92
• **Exhibitionism: the Burden of Taboos**	92

4 LOVE-MAKING POSITIONS

• **Variations on the Positions or 52 Ways of Making Love**	97

5 THE RISKS OF BREAK-UP

- **Opening the Dialogue** 197
  - *Showing mutual respect and accepting differences* 200
  - *Knowing how to take the initiative* 201

- **Jealousy: Love's Poison** 203

- **Infidelity: Wounded Love** 207
  - *Emotional dissatisfaction* 207
  - *Sexual dissatisfaction* 207
  - *The need to prove one really exists* 208
  - *The whims of age* 209
  - *Taking advantage of others* 209
  - *Tit for tat* 209
  - *Should one admit to being unfaithful?* 210
  - *Some testimonies* 211

- **Sexual Weariness** 214
  - *Love on the hour* 215
  - *Exciting experiences* 215
  - *Sex games* 216
  - *Working too hard* 216

6 PLEASURE UNDER THREAT

- **Obsession with the Size of the Penis** 219
  - *Virility is not measured in centimetres* 220
  - *Increasing the size of the penis* 223

- **Premature Ejaculaton: A Sexual Problem that can be Cured** 223
  - *Some testimonies* 223
  - *The treatments* 226

- **Difficulties with Erection and Impotence** 228
  - *Sex therapy* 231
  - *Some testimonies* 232

- **The Premenstrual Syndrome: 77 per cent of Women Suffer from It** 235
  - *Some testimonies* 235

- **The Problems of Orgasm for a Woman** 237
  - *Dyspareunia: pain and not pleasure* 237
  - *Vaginism: refusing to make love* 237
  - *Frigidity: little or no pleasure* 238

7 THE COUPLE AND CONTRACEPTION

- **Natural Methods and Contraceptive Products** 243
  - *The pill and pills* 243
  - *The coil* 244
  - *The diaphragm* 245
  - *Spermicides* 246
  - *The condom* 246
  - *The temperature method* 247
  - *Withdrawal or coitus interruptus* 247
  - *Some testimonies* 248

8 LIFE AND LOVE AFTER FIFTY

- **Arriving at Middle Age** 253
  - *Some testimonies* 253
  - *What happens at menopause?* 254
  - *Men as well...* 256

- **Love after Fifty** 257
  - *Reactions of the male sexual organs* 258
  - *How women change* 258
  - *The difficult age* 259

- **Plants to Reawaken the Senses** 260
  - *More for the sexual tonic* 262
  - *Recipes for romantic occasions* 263

9 MEDICAL FILE

- **Problems for the Male** 267
  - *The male sexual hormones* 267
  - *Sperm* 268
  - *Phimosis* 269
  - *The prostate* 269
  - *Vasectomy* 270

- **Sexology and Gynaecology** 271
  - *The gynaecological examination* 271
  - *Ultra-sound examination* 272
  - *Laparoscopy* 272
  - *X-raying the uterus* 274
  - *The female sexual hormones* 275
  - *Drying of the vagina* 276

Lack of periods 276
Painful periods 277
Episiotomy 278
Fibroma 278
Ovarian cysts 279
Endometriosis 280
Osteoporosis 281
Ovariectomy 281
Female surgical sterilization 282
Hormonal skin patches 283

- The Couple and Sexual Health 283
Sexual hygiene 283
Tobacco and sexuality 284
Cholesterol and sexual health 285
The effect of certain medicines on sexuality 286
Excess alcohol and sexuality 286
Infections of the genital organs 287

10 SOME QUESTIONS AND ANSWERS 291

11 INDEX 300

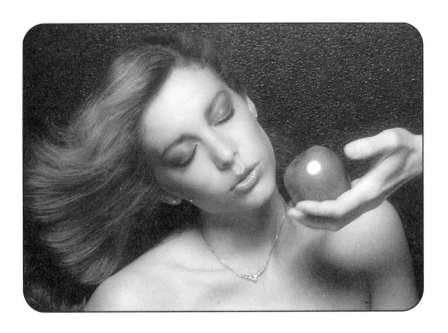

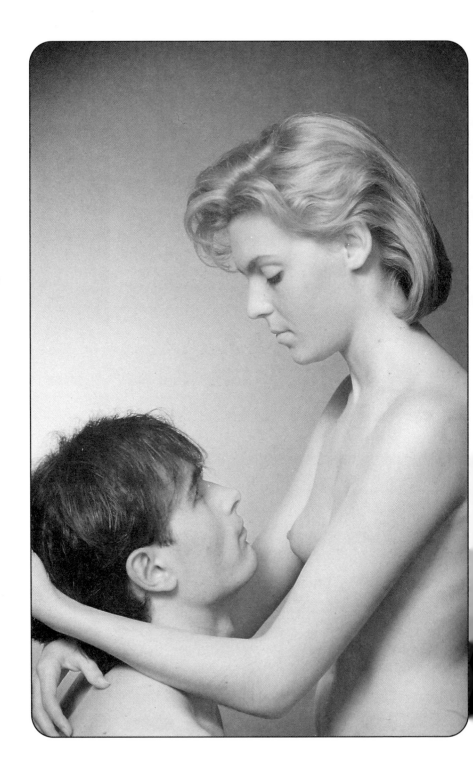

A MAN, A WOMAN: THE ENCOUNTER, THE DESIRE

·

Two people meet ... attracted to each other.
It is the beginning of love and desire.
The first amorous gestures ...
What happens in the heart and in the body ...

·

LOVE: THE HAPPINESS AND THE TEARS

Devotion, adoration, attachment, tenderness, desire ... all of these are part of love, as is happiness – and tears. Among the definitions to be found in the dictionary, perhaps the most appropriate would be: 'That feeling of attachment which is based upon difference of sex; the affection between lover and sweetheart'.

A man, a woman, the encounter ... Whether at the age of seventeen or sixty, something happens between two people, a flash, a sudden desire to get closer, to look into each other's eyes, to touch ... A warmth that fills head and body ... The absolute need to know this other person ...

This is the beginning of love, a great love, the kind of love one reads about in novels and sees on the screen. It is happiness at first sight. Neither can pass the other by. It is the moment when two people discover all the pleasures of love, from the first tender words of affection to the final outbursts of passion.

It is difficult to think of love without sensual harmony, except perhaps with the very young or the very old. According to Victor Hugo, "to love is to savour in the arms of a loved one the heaven that God put into our flesh".

At the cinema, as in real life, love stories always start off happily. But, as Marcel Proust pessimistically but also realistically observed: "In love, happiness is an abnormal state". People can love each other, adore each other... and tear each other apart. Jean Anouilh described the situation as follows: "To love each other is to struggle constantly against the millions of hidden forces we and the world create".

These hidden forces include, of course, the anxieties of everyday life – worries about money, family and work problems, health risks and so on. Perhaps Anouilh was exaggerating a little, but certainly everyone can make up their own list from personal experience.

So how can we battle against these hidden forces and save love? Through a deep internal bond within the relationship, mutual respect and a continually enriched sexual life. When a man and a woman share true love, together they develop a psychological and sensual maturity which provides the most solid of links.

"Love is also about always being concerned for the other." This quote from Marcel Achard is worth remembering, since it underlines the need to be unselfish. To preoccupy oneself with the well-being and pleasure of one's partner must be the concern of every couple.

Living together day after day can take the edge off a loving relationship if those involved fail to cherish it and allow themselves to behave in a way that will upset the other. This could involve being too domineering, letting parents or in-laws get in the way or spending too much time in front of the television. Failing to look after one's body or neglecting the way one dresses can also put pressure on a relationship, whether it be the man or the woman. Perhaps it is only a question of detail, but it can matter all the same.

Examples of bad or upsetting habits which one can acquire without even knowing it are numerous...

- Valerie, who feels the cold badly, wears two pullovers in bed. Her husband is put off by the idea of having to take them off before he cuddles her.
- Terry always watches television until the end of the last programme and Yvonne has to go to bed alone.
- Every evening Robert phones his mother just as the meal is about to be served and stays talking for ages.
- Peter walks around the house in pyjamas while Rose is smartly dressed.

Of course these are in themselves just little things, part of everyday life. But they can eventually destroy a relationship.

TAKING THE ROUGH WITH THE SMOOTH

Is there such a thing as a forever kind of love? Certainly. Everyone knows of couples who, after thirty years or more of marriage, still live happily together and continue to provide each other with affection and care. With such couples there is a special feeling of peace and happiness which comes from sharing life and its pleasures.

But who knows? Maybe they too have had their problems which we do not know about.

In fact it is rare, if not exceptional, that things always go smoothly – even in the best of worlds. And the world today is far from being ideal as far as protecting relationships is concerned.

The temptations of modern life provide a constant threat. Sometimes they concern money or possibly another person. Perhaps there are violent disagreements, although here at least true love can prevail and pardon.

Possibly the most serious is the sexual weariness that may set in as the years go by. This can lead to indifference and sometimes even aggression. As a result, the relationship is put under strain through reproaches and agonizing disputes.

Such confrontations can be avoided by tackling the reality head-on from the moment when the couple first senses a deterioration. Both must face up to the truth of the situation and search for mutual agreement on the desire to continue to live in harmony.

If the real desire is there, then love still exists and the relationship can be saved.

EXPRESSING LOVE IN LETTERS

Letters exchanged between those who love each other, but who are at the time apart, come straight from the heart. The words are spontaneous and the emotional ties are maintained.

There are plenty of examples to be found in both history and literature involving some of the great love affairs. The French in particular, with their tradition for full-blooded romance, never seem to be at a loss for words when it comes to expressing their innermost feelings.

Even if not everybody possesses the gift of such powerful expression, those who have suffered the loneliness of being separated from their loved ones will certainly be touched by many of the passages.

During the forty years of their passionate relationship, Juliette Drouet wrote more than eighteen thousand letters to Victor Hugo. Here are several extracts from their correspondence.

- "I love you because I love you. I love you because it would be impossible for me not to love you. I love you without thinking, without any hidden motive, without reason – good or bad. I love you with all my heart, with all my soul, with every possible way there is to love. You must believe it, because it's true! . . ."
- "My dear adorable one, nineteen years ago to the day you left my

embrace for the first time and, for the first time also, I suffered this terrible emptiness and deep sadness that I have always suffered since, every time you are separated from me. Since the very first day, my eyes have followed you as far as they could see you and my heart has followed your heart everywhere. My Victor, my beloved, my sublime adorable one, I have loved you since the first time I saw you and my whole body thrills to the touch of your dear little hand. To me you are like a flame that fires my heart and lights up my soul. I love you more than I can tell you, more than all the world. I love you, I love you, I love you."
- "As soon as you are gone, I don't live any more, I don't think any more, I don't hope any more. I want you and I suffer. I also fear more than death our return to that hideous Paris, where there is nothing for lovers who love each other like we do. Nothing, neither sunshine, nor hope – that sunshine of love, nothing but rain, suspicion and jealousy, the three blackest, saddest and coldest of plagues, which strike at the body and the soul.

"Oh! I suffer, my Toto, as much as I love you, it is true, my poor adorable one, and it is always so when you are not with me."

Another example of the exchange of passionate letters comes from Napoleon Bonaparte, writing to Josephine . . .
- "I wake up full of you. Your picture and the memory of yesterday's intoxicating evening have given me no rest at all. Sweet, incomparable Josephine, what strange effect you have on my heart! Are you angry? Do I see you sad? Are you worried? My soul is so touched with grief that there is no peace at all for your friend. But is it then better for me, while surrendering to the deep feeling that controls me, to draw from your lips, from your heart, a flame which burns me . . ."
- "I have not spent a single day without loving you or a single night without holding you tight in my arms. I have not drunk a single cup of tea without cursing the glory and ambition that keep me far away from the love of my life. In the midst of the action, at the head of my troops, while touring the camps, my adorable Josephine is alone in my heart, occupying my soul, consuming my thoughts . . ."

Mirabeau, a brilliant speaker who wanted to defend the monarchy at the time of the French Revolution, was madly in love with a young woman called Sophie de Monnier. The letters he wrote to her are famous – and rightly so – like this one:
- "Trust and rare tenderness seem to me the real signs of passion. That is how it is with me and I hope you will allow me to say that there is not another so tender; save only yours, of course, so

that you do not sulk. Yes, my dear Sophie, I do believe that from the bottom of my soul. Our hearts were made just for each other; you alone have been able to make me faithful, even amorous, because you must not think, oh my friend, that I have never known love before you. The fever of my senses is no more related to the ecstasies that you instill in me than there can be comparison between you and the women I respected before we were married. I have told you so a hundred times: your tongue, scented when it wanders over my lips, excites me a thousand times more than I ever was by the ultimate pleasure I gained in the arms of another woman. It is a triumph you will never know how to appreciate, my friend, but one that comforts me, to have for so long flattered other beauties, in order to prove to myself what a difference there is between the desires of nature and those of love, and that, as a result, I have loved only you . . ."

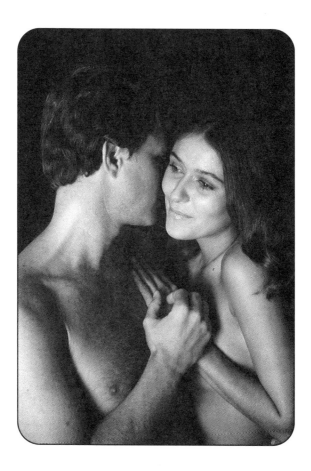

THE SENSUAL WEALTH OF YOUR BODY

DISCOVERING YOUR FEMININITY

Only in the privacy of the bathroom or bedroom can you really discover your body. Don't be modest. You can and must study every detail and familiarise yourself with your anatomy. Make sure that there is no risk of anyone disturbing you and that you have some time to yourself. Get undressed completely and look at yourself in the mirror.

First the front. What are you breasts like? You think they are too small and that depresses you because you dream of having full breasts like those of some of the film or television stars you see.

That is the time to think about such stars as Jane Birkin and Charlotte Rampling and be satisfied because age will not spoil your breasts, the skimpiest of bathing costumes will always look decent on you and you will not need to wear a bra except when you want to dress up or wear pretty underwear.

Are your breasts well-developed, pointed in the shape of a pear or round like an apple? In any case, they represent a feminine symbol regarded as a major asset of seduction.

With young women, the perfect balance of hormones assures firm breasts. Age and child-bearing can, to a greater or lesser degree, cause the breasts to sag. This can be prevented by taking the appropriate exercise, wearing a suitable size bra, having cold showers and frequently using special creams.

If, when you have examined yourself objectively in front of the mirror, you are still convinced that your breasts are too big and too soft and you feel 'abnormal' to the point that your psyche and sex life are being seriously affected, you can resort to having plastic surgery.

The preliminary consultation will enable the surgeon to decide on the merits of your need, to explain what the operation involves, including its results and after-effects, and to help you decide whether you wish to go ahead.

Having looked carefully at and assessed your breasts, now touch and caress them gently, pinch your nipples lightly and run your fingers all round the areole.

The breasts are one of the principal erogenous zones of a woman's body. You will very probably feel pleasure and will notice the nipples becoming erect as your breasts turn pink and swell. This is what happens during the sexual act as excitement grows.

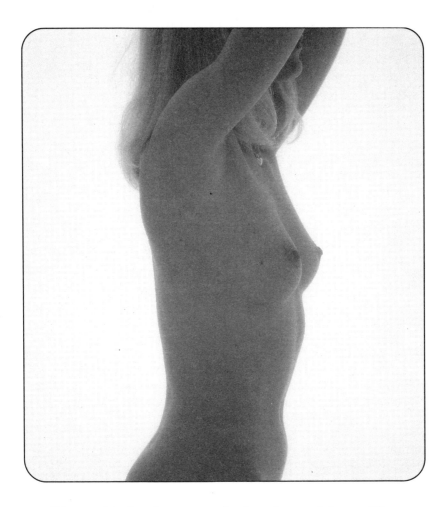

The pubis is also named after the goddess of love

Now look down at the triangle of hairs that covers your pubis, also more poetically known as the Mount of Venus. Yes, these hairs are the same colour as the hair on your head and your eyebrows and, like them, they can turn white with age.

The pubic hairs, which are generally curly, sometimes frizzy and more or less plentiful among women, can spread up as far as the belly-button and down the inside of the thighs. They are much appreciated by certain men, who find them an erotic attraction.

But if this hairy forest does not please you, it is perfectly easy to have it removed, preferably by a specialist beautician. And there are those who prefer to be completely hairless to simulate the condition of youth.

In fact the pubic fleece has its purpose. Having protected the genital organs since human life began, it preserves the sexual odours, specific to each individual, that the most fastidious hygienic care and use of perfumes and deodorants do not succeed in getting rid of completely.

This *odor di femina* has a really erotic influence to which many men are susceptible and which is often a great source of excitement in love-play.

The vulva, a universe to explore

Now have a look at the most intimate parts of your body. Sit down comfortably with your legs apart and, with the help of a small mirror, study your external genital organs, collectively known as the vulva. This is made up of the outer and inner lips, the clitoris, the urinary opening and the entrance to the vagina.

The two outer lips start from the base of the Mount of Venus and finish about two or three centimetres from the anus. They are hairy and generally pinky-brown and sometimes almost chestnut in colour. By separating the outer lips, you will uncover the inner lips – again, two of them – which are pink, damp and hairless. Their edges can be either smooth or serrated.

The clitoris, an essential organ of pleasure

At the top of the inner lips you will find the clitoris, the essential organ of female pleasure. It is a protuberance of flesh of varying size according to the individual whose root, measuring two or three centimetres, is sunk into the tissues.

The clitoris has often been compared with a penis in miniature since, like this organ, it comprises a stem and a gland, a sort of small round cylindrical button which protects a hood formed where the two inner lips meet.

When the clitoris, which is made up of erectile tissues and nerve endings, is stimulated by being stroked or during sexual intercourse, it swells up, becomes erect and frees itself from its hood.

Create the experience yourself by exciting it with your fingers. You will feel an excitement which will increase until, if you continue stroking it, you reach a state of orgasm – just by the simple stimulation of the clitoris.

If you look below the clitoris, you will see the urinary opening through which your urine passes. It is linked to the bladder by the urethra canal. Although not a sexual organ, it is very sensitive.

The vagina and its mysteries

Still holding the outer and inner lips apart, look at the entrance of the vagina, an opening of about five centimetres in diameter. Slide your finger inside. You will find it is hot (37°C) and moist.

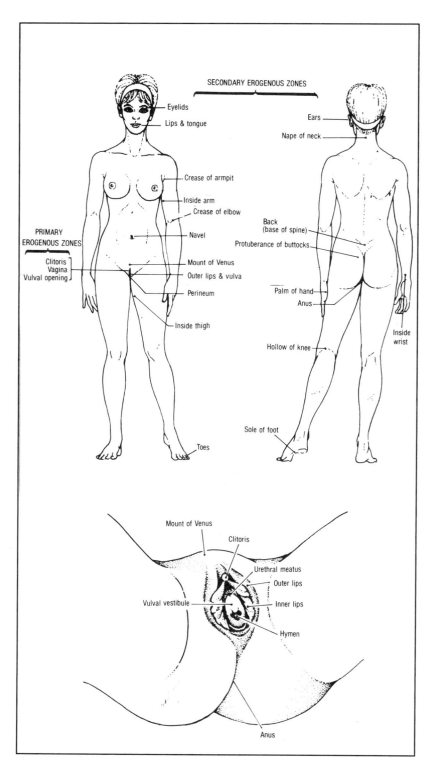

You can only examine the entrance of the vagina, which opens on to a fleshy passage, whose elasticity you can appreciate by pushing in one or two fingers. This will cause the muscles in the pelvis to contract. You will feel the vagina tightening around your fingers.

You should also know that inside the vulva there are some invisible glands, each of which has a precise role to play.

The sweat glands, which are in the roots of the pubic hair, secrete a fluid with a specific odour. The sebaceous glands in the 'cushion' of the Mount of Venus secrete a fat, the sebum, which lubricates the pilosity.

There are two other sets of glands which begin the lubrication of the vagina, essential for penetration and copulation. These are the Skene glands, near the urinary opening, and the Bartholin glands, in the outer lips near the anus.

That explains the external genital organs, the only ones that you are really able to see. However, you should also know about the internal genital organs, since they too play a part in your sexuality.

Let us first go back to the vagina, the passage running from the vulva to the uterus, which normally measures about ten centimetres outside sexual intercourse. Made up of elastic fibres, the vagina can lengthen to as much as fifteen centimetres during intercourse and expand to about five centimetres to accommodate the size of your partner's penis. And finally, at the time of childbirth, the vagina swells out to facilitate the passage of the baby's head (on average ten centimetres in diameter).

Innervated for the first third of its length, making this part particularly sensitive, the vagina is lined with a fine mucous membrane. It is always pink in colour, regardless of the woman's race.

The walls of the vagina are always extremely active. They get rid of dead cells and, at the same time, ensure perpetual regeneration. They also produce a kind of whitish coating, whose acidity protects the vagina from harmful bacteria. And finally, through the influence of stimulation and sexual excitement, they secrete a lubricating liquid without which copulation would not only be painful but would also risk inflaming the fragile mucous membrane.

At the entrance of the vagina you will find the hymen, a thin membrane in the middle of which is a small opening for the discharge during periods and vaginal secretions.

An intact hymen is regarded as the symbol and proof of virginity, the first sexual experience – the deflowering – being deemed to have torn it, thus provoking profuse bleeding. But plenty of young virgins have torn their hymen simply in the course of playing sport.

Once broken, under whatever circumstances, the hymen will appear as small irregular indentations around the entrance of the vagina.

Can you touch your hymen with the end of your finger? It is not easy because, whether you are still a virgin or you have already had sexual intercourse, this membrane does not always obstruct the vagina. Its form varies from one woman to another. It can be in the shape of a ring or a crescent or, indeed, be riddled with little holes. It is also possible that you may have little or no hymen. As for seeing it, that can only be done through gynaecological examination.

The uterus, a masterpiece of nature

At the bottom of the vagina the cervix opens out. This organ, about two centimetres long, forms the lower part of the uterus and is shaped like an inverted pear. It contains a small opening which allows the spermatozoons to enter the uterus and the blood to escape during periods.

From the fourteenth day of the cycle, the cervix produces a mucus which resembles and has the same consistency as the white of an egg. This mucus helps the spermatozoons to move towards the uterus and the Fallopian tubes. It equally plays a part in lubricating the vagina.

The uterus itself is made up of three superimposed layers of muscular fibres which form a strong and extremely resistant tissue. With women who have never borne a child, it is about six centimetres wide and stretches up to eight or nine centimetres for those who have.

The internal wall is about ten millimetres thick at the bottom of the uterus and between twelve and fifteen millimetres elsewhere. Between the walls there is a cavity about seven centimetres high and three-and-a-half centimetres wide where the foetus grows. The elasticity of these walls is such that, at the height of growth, the volume of the cavity will have increased tenfold.

On both sides of the uterus there are two thin tubes which connect with the ovaries. These are the Fallopian tubes along which the ovule (or egg) travels to join up with the spermatozoon which impregnates it.

The ovaries, the feminine sexual glands, are positioned under the tubes. Two in number and the size of a pigeon's egg, these glands have a double function – the production of the ovule, one a month, and the feminine sexual hormones, the progesterone and the oestrogens.

These hormones intervene not only in the cycle, the function of reproduction, but also in the physical feminine characteristics such as the shape of the body, the breasts, the voice and even in the erotic appetite and physiological modifications which contribute to the success of the sexual act.

Understand yourself

All these mechanisms, all this alchemy can seem a little complicated. But to know about it all will help you to understand better the reactions of your body.

You will know, for example, that if your lubrication becomes more profuse from the fourteenth day of your cycle, then this is because the cervix has started to produce some mucus; that, during sexual intercourse, your vagina is going to adapt to the size of your partner's penis; and that, if you are pregnant, your uterus, the true birthplace of your child, will transform itself simultaneously and proportionately – from seven centimetres high and three-and-a-half centimetres wide to more than thirty centimetres by twenty to twenty-two.

Thank you, Mr Grafenberg

During the Forties, German gynaecologist Ernest Grafenberg discovered that women have in the vagina a small zone which, suitably stimulated, provokes intense sensations and leads to orgasms accompanied by the emission of a colourless and odourless liquid.

But it was not until the Eighties that some American researchers confirmed the existence of this zone, which they called the G Spot after its 'discoverer' – Dr Grafenberg. Thanks to their work, it was possible to locate this point very precisely – just behind the pubic bone in the outer wall of the vagina between the urine excretion canal and the base of the bladder. It is an organ the size of a small bean which trebles in volume under the effect of stimulation.

Do all women have a G Spot?

Well, after observations made on volunteers, it would appear that this is now confirmed. But certainly few women know of the existence of this source of pleasure.

Is it possible to touch one's G Spot?

Not very easily, since the organ lies deep in the vagina. Here is the best way of reaching it.

Get down on your knees, with your legs apart, and sit on your heels. Naturally, you need to be naked. Slide two fingers of one hand into your vagina and, with the palm of the other hand, press quite hard on the base of your stomach. Your fingers will reach the outer wall of the vagina where they must search for the spot at which they can begin to create the sensations. Under the effect of this excitement, the G Spot is going to grow in size and become obvious. Its prolonged stimulation will start an orgasm which those women who have succeeded in reaching it say is absolutely extraordinary.

There is no doubt that the gymnastics involved in such exploration demand time and plenty of patience. There are other, more simple ways of experiencing pleasure.

We should add that the orgasm achieved from the G Spot is accompanied by what certain sexologists have called a 'feminine ejaculation'. This is, in effect, a fluid in which analysis has revealed an enzyme that is equally found in the secretions of the man's prostate.

For the woman who has learned how to find and stimulate her G Spot, she can share the secret with her partner. Guided by her, he can stimulate it with one of his fingers in the precise place. Alternatively, during sexual intercourse, his erect penis can make contact with the G Spot. But this is only possible where the woman is astride the man or with backward penetration. By moving her pelvis, the woman will lead her partner simultaneously and appropriately to the sensations she will feel.

If you do not want to involve yourself in such experiences, refrain from discovering the G Spot, however it provides proof of vaginal pleasure and how the vagina is not 'insensitive' as people had for a long time considered.

The other sensitive pleasure spots

You adore eating oysters, biting into chocolate, tasting an old port. The pleasures of good eating mark out your life and that is your absolute right, just like the search for sensual pleasures which are a form of gormandizing otherwise referred to by sexologists as the erotic appetite.

The satisfaction of this appetite comes through the discovery of your body, which is the 'instrument' of your pleasure. You learn how to examine your genital organs and prove their sensitivity through caresses. These are the erogenous zones, so called after Eros, the god of love, and 'gene', which generates. When stimulated, these spots give birth to both desire and pleasure.

Your genital organs belong to the erogenous zones known as 'primary', although there are certainly others, unjustly called 'secondary' since they too are the source of infinite pleasure. You are going to explore these as well with the tips of your fingers. They are spread over roughly two square metres of the surface of your skin.

Gently touch your lips, the rim of your mouth; lightly caress your ears and your neck, on the nape and under the chin; move down as far as the armpits and linger in the folds of the inside of your arms. Softly pinch the point of your breasts and gently massage your nipples and areoles. The hollow of the elbows, knees and hands, the waistline, the navel and the area around it, the Mount of Venus, the wrists, the folds of the groin, the soles of the feet and the toes are all areas that offer a world of sensations.

In exploring for yourself these erogenous zones, you will certainly not experience as much pleasure as you would if they were caressed by your partner. But you will learn to recognise the degree of their sensitivity.

Do not forget that everyone is different and that not all women will react in the same way. Some, for example, will burst out laughing if one strokes the soles of their feet or their navel. It is therefore up to you to establish your own personal 'geography' and to guide your partner so that he will know your sensitive spots.

Have no qualms about seeming egoistic in seeking your own pleasure. The man you love and who loves you will be doubly satisfied because love is an exchange and you will know how to offer him as much as he gives you.

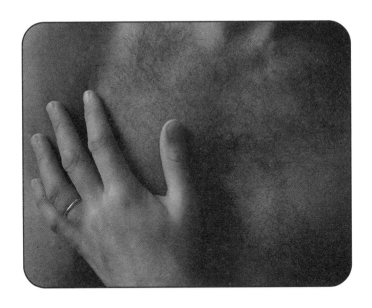

The erotic geography of your body

The great journey of exciting caresses passes through those parts of the body particularly sensitive to excitement – the erogenous zones.

While they are all catalogued by the sexologists, they do not react in the same way for every individual. Every woman has her own special spots. Their discovery lies with the couple through touches, caresses and kissing.

Those erogenous zones sensitive to caressing are indicated on the illustrations of the female body (*see page 19*). Try them on yourself and on your partner and, in your love-play, make the most of those that provide the greatest sensations.

DISCOVERING YOUR MALE VIRILITY

To arrive at obtaining and giving the maximum of pleasure, you must know your body well. Spend time studying it in all its detail and testing its reactions. Without false modesty and in front of a mirror where you can observe yourself from head to foot, examine yourself carefully and thoroughly.

The organ for sexual intercourse

Your eyes will, without doubt, in the first instance head straight for your most obvious masculine attributes – the penis and the scrotum.

The penis varies in length when it is 'resting' – while it is floppy – as well as when it is erect. We will be discussing the subject of the size of the penis in greater detail, since this is one of the male's constant preoccupations.

Of course, everyone knows that the penis is used for sexual intercourse. Round in shape and covered with a very fine skin, the colour of which varies from pink to brown depending on the individual, it hides inside a canal sixteen to twenty centimetres long known as the urethra, through which the urine passes – because it is linked to the bladder – or the sperm at the time of ejaculation. Such is the double function of the urethra, of which you can only see the tip, a small opening at the end of the penis, the urinary meatus.

What you cannot see is the inside of your penis, which comprises two cavities running along it on both sides and a third spongy formation, like tiny balloons made up of small cells which, under the effect of sexual excitement, fill up with blood and make the penis swell and then harden. The skin smooths out as the penis straightens and points upwards, forming a more or less acute angle with the stomach, according to the degree of excitement and one's age.

You can experiment with that yourself in front of the mirror by stroking your penis and creating provocative images in your mind.

At the end of the penis there is a swelling. This is the glans, with very fine pink skin, very sensitive, covered by a fold of skin –

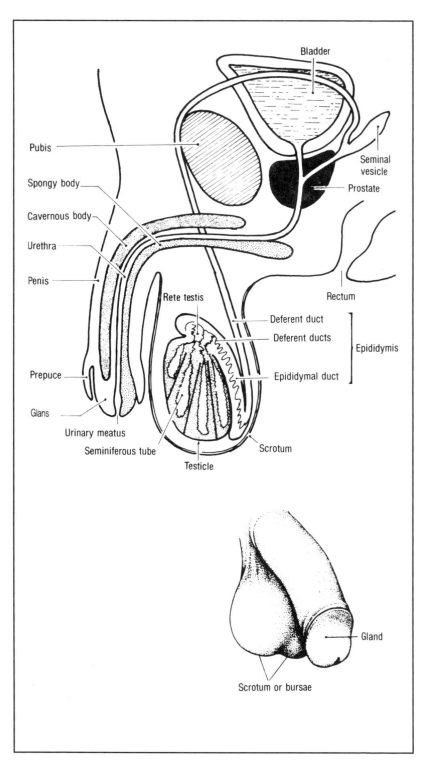

the prepuce or foreskin – and with its interior held by a small piece of skin known as the bride.

While the penis is at rest, the foreskin covers up the glans. At the time of erection, it slides like a sheath and releases – or exposes – the glans.

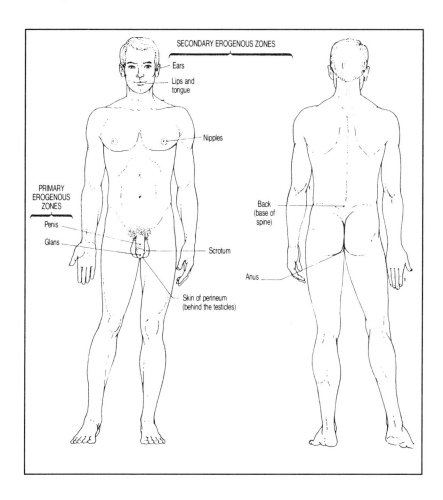

Sometimes it happens that the foreskin is too tight to slide over the glans or the bride too short to allow a full erection. This is known as a phimosis, which makes sexual intercourse painful and sometimes even impossible. In such instances it is necessary to have a small operation, which involves either cutting the bride or removing part or all of the foreskin.

This operation, which is simple, quick and without risk, is in fact the circumcision practised in certain countries for reasons of hygiene and obligatory in the Jewish and Muslim religions.

The testicles – veritable little factories

Behind the penis – and hanging a little lower – you will find the scrotum, kinds of bags of wrinkled, light brown skin containing the testicles. These are the male sex glands. You can feel them through the skin of the scrotum.

There are, in fact, two of them, in the form of small eggs about five centimetres long and three centimetres thick. They are mobile and very sensitive.

Do not be alarmed to find that they are not always at the same height or of the same size.

These testicles are real little factories. They produce the male hormones which are responsible for the virile appearance of the male (muscles, hairiness, voice, etc . . .) and produce the spermatozoons, the fertilizing elements of the sperm.

If you cause an erection of your penis, you will notice that your scrotum will swell, harden and rise and the skin will loose its wrinkles.

Perhaps you have already had the occasion to notice that under very bracing, cold conditions (an icy shower, for example), your scrotum will contract while under hot conditions it will soften and hang down.

These contrasting effects are explained by the reaction of a muscle in the skin of the scrotum to extreme temperatures.

Between the penis and the anus is the perineum, which consists of a band of muscles that support your genital organs.

From the triangle to the pubic diamond

Now have a look at the hairs on your body, which you can find all over the body but particularly on the pubis. Here the hairs will have started to push through at puberty in the form of a triangle, as with the female, then split up in the form of a diamond.

They are curly and frizzy, the same colour as the hair on your head, streaking white with age, and are more or less prolific depending on the individual.

At the same time as your pubic hairs begin to appear, so do the beard, the hairs under your armpits and those on your chest.

It is often said that excessive hairiness is a sign of virility. There is no connection here.

Sensitive nipples

Yes, men do have breasts – or, more precisely, mammary glands. But whereas with women, under the effect of specific sexual hormones, these develop to a very noticeable extent, with men one hardly sees these since they are usually very small and surrounded by an areole which can sometimes be quite hairy.

So touch your nipples, pinch them, tickle them, at the same time imagining it is a woman caressing them. You will feel them harden under your fingers, expand and become erect, while sending waves of excitement through your body.

Too many men – and women, for that matter – are ignorant of the fact that the male breasts are an extremely sensitive erogenous zone which should not be overlooked in the foreplay to lovemaking.

What more can you see in front of your mirror once you have discovered your external genital organs in all their detail?

Nothing else. But you should know that from each of your testicles runs a thin tube, the deferent duct, which measures between thirty and fifty centimetres in length.

After a long course across the scrotum and the abdomen, each duct circles the bladder, rejoins the seminal vesicle (or spermary) and finally runs into the prostate.

This is a gland found at the base of the bladder, whose shape resembles that of a chestnut and whose volume varies with age, doubling or even tripling in size by the time one reaches one's sixties.

Invisible from the outside, the prostate can only be felt through the rectum, allowing doctors to appraise its shape and consistency. The urethra runs inside its entire length.

The gland produces the prostatic fluid whose function is to dilute the spermatozoons carried from the testicles through the deferent ducts in order to make the sperm. At the moment of ejaculation, it contracts and empties like a sponge, thus contributing to the release of the sperm.

The prostate is crowned by two elongated glands, the seminal vesicles, which measure about four centimetres long and are as thick as a little finger. They produce a sticky secretion, rich in fructose, a sugar that is indispensible for the nutrition of the spermatozoons.

TEST YOUR EROTIC SENSIBILITY

Look again in the mirror to discover which points on your body are more especially sensitive to pleasure. We call these the erogenous zones.

You have already tried caressing your penis and nipples. You have noticed that they stiffen up and become hard. Now search out with your fingers those other spots that respond to stimulation.

With the tip of your index finger, gently stroke your saliva-moistened lips, follow the outline of your ears, lightly rub the nape of your neck, the inside of your thighs, the scrotum, the perineum and the anal region.

It is up to you to take note of your sexual reactions to these touches. With some there may be little response, while with others you will experience varying degrees of excitement. Also imagine that it is your partner who is lavishing all these caresses on you with her hands, her mouth and her tongue.

In this way you can test your erotic sensibility. And, when it comes to the foreplay, guide your companion towards those zones where real pleasure is born.

PLEASURE ON ONE'S OWN

The practice of arousing pleasure by exciting one's genital parts by hand – called auto-eroticism or masturbation – was for a long time considered unhealthy, even dangerous. Some of the worst effects attributed to it included neuralgia, incontinence, impaired sight, deafness and insanity.

Today such tales have happily been buried. And the study by sexologists throughout the world has shown that masturbation during childhood is the best introduction to successful erotic experiences as an adult.

Even at the tenderest of ages, babies gain pleasure from touching their sexual organs. This natural and instinctive gesture recurs in childhood and later in adolescence. It is rare to find those who do not practise auto-eroticism.

Despite this, some parents still get upset by it and even go so far as to try and ban it and threaten punishment. For them we must repeat that there is nothing to fear now or for the future from children indulging in such pleasures on their own.

Parents must turn a blind eye and not run the risk of making their children feel in any way guilty or giving them a complex that could remain with them throughout their future sex life.

Take the following case history.

"One night I caught my seven-year-old daughter 'touching herself'. I had gone into her bedroom about an hour after she went to sleep. I switched on the bedside lamp to look at her sleeping and was rearranging the covers when I saw her little hand resting on her sexual organ. I felt a sudden pang of revulsion.

"I went downstairs to tell my husband and said I would give her a stiff reprimand in the morning. He smiled at me and replied gently: 'And you never did that when you were a child?' I couldn't deny it and decided not to scold her.

"Some time later I met the pediatrician who looked after my daughter. I asked him if there was any cause for concern. He fully reassured me that there wasn't."

This 29-year-old mother, who with her husband's help chose to accept what had initially shocked her, provides a good example

of the attitude parents must adopt in similar situations.
It is incredible to think that in the 19th century all sorts of gadgets were invented for tying up children's hands to prevent them from touching their sexual organs and masturbating! The practice of self-induced sexual pleasure is most commonly carried out by adults – and for a variety of reasons. Maybe it is because the individual has yet to experience sex as a couple. Perhaps it is to make up for a partner's temporary absence. It could even be to fulfil those desires that one's companion does not satisfy.

However, masturbation need not always be a self-induced pleasure. It can also be part of a couple's love-play, whether carried out simultaneously by each one on the other to achieve a shared excitement or one that is reciprocated in turn.

According to a recent report on the sexual behaviour of Europeans, masturbation was practised by married men as follows: 80 per cent of 20-29-year-olds, 77 per cent of 30-49-year-olds and 60 per cent of those over 50. And for married women the figures were 23 per cent, 19 per cent and 15 per cent respectively.

Masturbating techniques are most commonly manual: an up-and-down movement of the hand on the man's penis and, for the woman, stimulation of the clitoris with the finger and stroking of the vulva.

The pleasure to be gained from such experiences can mount as one's erotic life evolves and as each individual learns how to achieve the ultimate orgasm.

In all cases and for all ages, masturbation feeds on fantasies (*see Chapter 3*).

You may sometimes hear people talking about onanism as the equivalent of masturbation. Well, onanism is in fact the practice of coitus interruptus (interrupted copulation).

The origins of this go back 2000 years, when Onan refused to obey the Levitical law which obliged him to provide his brother's widow with an heir. In order not to make the woman pregnant, he used coitus interruptus. As punishment, Onan was struck down by a thunderbolt.

From what is, no doubt, just a biblical legend, people drew the conclusion that not to use semen to procreate was a sin. And, by extending the argument, it was also considered a sin to waste semen by masturbating.

The fact remains that a certain unrest over this practice continues to exist. Those who freely discuss their sexual exploits remain discreet about this particular habit.

Auto-eroticism is rarely a subject about which people confide, save perhaps among adolescents who want to compare their first sexual experiences with those of their friends.

As a final comment, masturbation is neither reprehensible nor harmful. But in adult life it should be used to enrich the love between two people and must not become a substitute for sex with a partner.

BODY LANGUAGE

The body has a language. It talks. Every movement sends out a message. You do not have to speak if you want to express a feeling of desire, affection, love or, for that matter, distaste.
Let's take a few examples.
Karen, who is 18, is at a wedding. Among the guests she notices a boy walking confidently around in a way that attracts her attention. She moves towards him, unaware of the fact that she has herself adopted an air of seduction. Her step is measured, her head is slightly hung to one side, her mouth reveals half a smile and her eyes sparkle. For the moment there are no signs of reaction from the boy whom she does not even know, except that his name is Alan.

When Karen finally catches up with him, she gently jostles past him to get to the buffet – an excellent pretext to be noticed.

A quick glance from the boy, whose assessment is as rapid as hers was (this girl has style and charm), an engaging smile and a convenient stretch of the arm to reach for a drink for his new-found companion.

Not a single word has been spoken. Yet Karen has already realised that Alan is not indifferent towards her. And, for his part, Alan has demonstrated by his reactions that he has got the message and that he is ready to respond.

In all this, there has not been a hint of open provocation or misplaced gestures, but simply body signals which have aroused a mutual attraction between the two young people.

Philip and Marion, both 20 and fellow law students, see each other several times a week at college. Marion is always in a hurry, arriving late and rushing off afterwards, and thus particularly elusive.

During lectures, Philip's eyes never leave her. Winking, raising his eyebrows and staring openly or through half-closed eyelids at the young girl, he tries to catch her eye. The message is unmistakeable. Only a few metres separate them, enough to provide Marion with some protection without putting her totally out of reach.

Finally, one morning, she turns and throws back her head as she runs her hand through her long black hair. The gesture is spontaneous, but the intention quite clear. Philip knows he has won the first round.

In such situations, gestures and signs can produce their own silent conversations and every body movement can be symbolic.

A man sitting in a classically laid-back position, leaning comfortably on the arm of a chair, one leg folded across the knee of the other, indicates his readiness to communicate, but also suggests an even greater opportunity – a willingness to respond to an emotional or sensual approach, often not fully recognised or appreciated by the opposite sex.

In the same way, a man leaning against a wall with his legs apart and his hands in his pocket is giving out the message that he wants to make contact.

In contrast, a woman sitting with her legs crossed and arms folded is quite clearly not trying to communicate with the opposite sex. In another, all too obvious example, she will give out quite the opposite signal if she takes a man by the arm or touches some part of his clothing to assess its quality or if, sitting cross-legged, she allows him to catch a glimpse of her underwear or bare flesh.

All contact postures are very significant. Sitting side by side or opposite one another with knees brushing and arms on the shoulder represent clearly decipherable advances.

As the next stage on from this kind of situation, one moves into the realms of seduction – the deliberate and often even calculated intention to arouse the sexual instincts of one's companion.

If, as has often been claimed, women are masters of this art, then men are certainly not lacking in such skills. Each can play with speech, use intonation in the voice, smile, make open advances and express through words and gestures the attraction felt for another.

Everyone plays their own game and makes their own rules. Suggestive looks, hand-stroking, soft words or, equally, feigned indifference and carefully calculated aggression are all well-used methods of stimulating a new relationship one wants to develop.

Carol, who is 23, met Paul at a friend's place. She was immediately attracted to him. He was laid-back, his voice was slightly rough and he had a short black beard. She began to put on the charm, but to no avail. Paul clearly preferred to talk about cars with a friend. Irritated by this, Carol quickly found a way of attracting his attention. She sarcastically asked Paul if he had lost his razor, at the same time stroking his beard and then the back of his neck.

Under the pretext of getting out her handkerchief, she then leant forward, pushing out her bust. The low neckline gave him every chance to see her breasts, which were scantily covered in white lace. Grabbing hold of Paul to lift herself back up, Carol stumbled and found herself in the arms of a man who had well and truly fallen into her trap and who, in the end, was delighted to be there.

In order to achieve her objectives in the first stage of what could become a really emotional and sexual relationship, Carol put her sex appeal to work. First of all, her self-confidence enabled her to go on the attack. She was able to demonstrate her sensuality by stroking Paul's beard and the back of his neck. She used verbal communication in order to surprise him, then made up for this act of aggression by letting him see her breasts – her femininity.

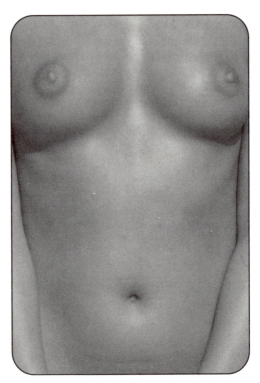

AIDS TO SEDUCTION

Essentially these are clothes, jewellery, make-up and perfume – a whole panoply to match the fashion, your personal taste and the desire to assert your own personality in your own way. Let's look at some of the most classic items that can be used in the process of seduction.

Take gloves, for example, and the way of slipping them on and peeling them off in a sensual fashion. Who can ever forget Rita Hayworth, in the famous film *Gilda*, removing her long black gloves finger by finger? It was a real striptease, immodest and at the same time elegant.

Tight sweaters that highlight the contours of the chest, wide belts that hold in the waist, mini-skirts that reveal virtually all one's legs, well-stretched black tights ending mid-thigh, stiletto heels or flat ones like those of a ballerina, evocative of youthful innocence, are all ways of looking to please.

Lace and see-through materials play the same role. Jewellery is irresistible to the eye. And make-up gives lips that 'kiss me' look, highlights eyes and produces an air of mystery and fascination.

But the panoply of seduction is not exclusively feminine. Men seek in their clothes a form of virility – jackets with broad shoulders, fitted jeans, splashes of bright or pastel colours, luminous prints and a thousand and one pocket items and scarves and ties, sometimes even printed with feminine designs.

If it is rare to see men wearing make-up, there is nevertheless no shortage of beauty products, including make-up foundations and creams, whose sales increase every year. Hair lotions, aftershave and other similar cosmetics are generally used by men of all ages. Increasingly now one sees rings, chains and bracelets being worn by men whose virility could not possibly be in doubt. And as for perfume, this is certainly used by members of both sexes.

The power of smell

From the earliest days of man, of all the five senses smell played the most important role in sexual attraction. Ignorance about hygiene left bodies with their natural odours, sweat and other secretions, to which those primitive humans who were our distant ancestors reacted like animals.

This is in stark contrast to the present day, where showers, baths, soap, lotions, cosmetics and deodorants have become very much part of everyday life. We do everything possible to disguise or completely get rid of our body odours and replace them with perfumes most often based on chemical products.

Nevertheless, despite all our efforts to battle against nature, it strikes back in the form of different substances we give off which release an odour. We do not smell this, but subconsciously it is noticed by others and amounts to a signal of sexual attraction.

Such substances, which are called pheromones, are secreted through glands and influence sexuality in a way that remains a mystery. One thing of which there is scientific evidence is that we have a smell memory lying dormant within us which a perfume or odour can arouse.

Thus the smell of cut hay may stir up memories of a holiday romance, a specific perfume may remind us of a woman we remember who wore it or sweat may recall a sporty person we once knew. One can cite plenty of examples like this where individuals react to certain smells. Whether positive or negative, this reaction is instinctive and almost inevitable.

Some women love to bury their face in their partner's armpit after making love, while others find such smells of 'animal' sweat disagreeable. For a number of men, the female sexual organ gives off a blend of odours that they find madly exciting. In fact, it is rare to find those who would deny their exotic power.

As well as natural smells, one must add those that one chooses in the form of eau de toilette and different perfumes. They all form part of the panoply of seduction, for men as well as for women. Equally, one must never overdo it, since too much artificial scenting can be off-putting.

GETTING RID OF COMPLEXES

Publicity, newspapers, cinema and television all depict images of beautiful, slim young women and strong, muscular, elegant men. But such media stereotypes hardly reflect the reality of everyday life.

Certainly girls today know how to look pretty and equally boys to look attractive. But not everyone has the shape or physique of a film or television star and a lot suffer from a feeling of inhibition which can make any kind of sentimental or sexual approach difficult, if not impossible.

"I am 18 years old", writes Helen. "I live in a small seaside town on the South Coast. During the summer, I go swimming early in the morning with my two sisters before starting work and when there is no-one else on the beach. I don't like to be seen in a bathing costume because I have enormous breasts.

"One day my brother told me in front of a friend of his: 'With these balloons there's no fear of you drowning!' That hurt me deeply and now I am always afraid that someone is going to laugh at my chest. I wear large, sloppy sweaters to cover it up and I avoid boys' groping hands at all costs."

For Virginia, the problem is that her nose is too long and her body is too small. As for Pauline, she believes her glasses make her look ugly and that she is incapable of pleasing any man because she is overweight.

Plenty of people suffer from an inferiority complex of one sort or another that condemns them to a self-inflicted solitude. This in turn prevents them from blossoming out.

For its part, the male sex is not exempt from this lack of self-confidence, which can very quickly prove a serious handicap in relationships with the opposite sex.

Whatever the shortcomings you think you have, learn to accept them and even take advantage of them. Make sure you know yourself well and appreciate your qualities so that others will appreciate them too. So you have acne. But you are unbeatable at tennis. The acne will take care of itself. Your championship strokes will attract their own attention. Mark was overweight, but he spoke French like a native. It was up to him to go on a diet. But his perfect knowledge of a foreign language would enable him to get a good job.

Beauty is not the only prerequisite for seducing the opposite sex. Everyone has something that can bring pleasure to others and must learn to exploit it. There is no lack of examples of great seducers who were bald, of adored women who were short-sighted or plump ones who ravaged men's hearts, of small men whose progress through life was littered with successful relationships with women. They had made the effort to ignore their physical shortcomings and make the most of their talents, of which everyone is naturally blessed, and do their best to develop them. Their reward: pleasure, love and being loved.

In an article in *Elle* magazine some years ago on the subject of seduction, the young novelist Alexandre Jardin wrote: "One needs talent to cultivate the art of being open while at the same time retaining an element of mystery, of always being someone else while at the same time remaining oneself, to seize each precious moment when one risks being buried in inertia, to be amazed each time the sun rises, to tease the others while at the same time making up to them."

FLIRTING: ONE STEP TOWARDS ADULT LOVE

Flirting involves a sentimental but sexually superficial relationship within well-established limits – a game with subtle rules.

In present-day society, it is almost unthinkable that a man of any age would make a direct proposition to a young girl, such as: "I like you a lot. Let's make love together." Custom demands that you do not go rushing straight in, but always start with gentle advances and a little flirtation.

A sentimental relationship, especially among adolescents and more particularly with girls, usually begins with normal friendship and then develops into something more amorous. And in adolescence a physical relationship marks the dawning of sexuality, the need for two people to get to know each other better.

A superficial relationship is most often a fleeting one and those who spend their time constantly flirting are unlikely to settle down and marry.

A more sincere, yet well-defined relationship allows, within the rules of the game, for kissing, caressing and touching but draws the line at actual love-making. One should know when to stop. And, in the heat of the moment, this is not always easy.

"I was 16 and he was 17 when we began flirting together," Carol admitted. "First we kissed each other and then he started to slide his hands under my pullover to stroke my breasts. That was very pleasant. Then he put his hands up my skirt to rub my vagina. Finally he pushed in one finger, two fingers ... I felt all hot inside.
"One day, he took my hand and put it on his penis. It was large and hard ... I did what he asked me. I stroked it. Then he wanted to go further. He wanted to make love.
"All that took place in some small woods in the country during the holidays. I was afraid of what was going to happen. I knew I didn't have to do it. So I ran off. I have since flirted with other boys, but never all the way."

Carol knew the price of her virginity and its symbolic value, which she had not lost despite her moral liberation. And, contrary to what a lot of parents believe, adolescents do limit themselves to physical acts of affection and share certain, sometimes intense, pleasures without indulging in the sexual act.

Flirting exists equally among adults. It is the display of a mutual desire which social or moral custom prevents us from taking to its natural conclusion.

Secret then open kissing, touching and caressing ... much pleasure is gained from those moments of real affection and love that inevitably lead to one partner trying to persuade the other to go the whole way. Perhaps it is the woman who refuses because they are already engaged and she does not want to spoil the relationship before the marriage. Equally it might be the man, who fears for his freedom and is having second thoughts about the engagement.

Claudia had been married for six years. She loved her husband Jack. They got on very well together in every respect. At work, Giles made eyes at her day after day. Naturally she was not insensitive to the fact that she was being admired and fancied. And where was the harm in having coffee or lunch with him or being taken home in his car?
As a matter of fact, it was in the car that Claudia accepted his initial kisses, the prelude to a mildly flirtatious relationship. But when Giles suggested that she came back to his flat, she refused, suddenly aware of the seriousness of a real affair and the consummation of an infidelity that would have very real consequences on the couple's future.

The case of Dennis is different. Twenty-eight years old and single, he enjoyed few adventures with women – and those he had were always brief affairs – and he never got attached.

Then he met Celia, an 18-year-old, who was to turn his life upside down. She gave him a lot of pleasure and he in turn thought he was in love with her. She was happy to flirt with him. She got the taste for it. And she had even decided to take the plunge and live with him. She talked about their happiness together, about marriage. But suddenly Dennis panicked at the idea of being trapped, of losing his precious freedom. He chose his freedom.

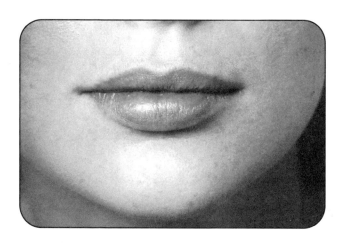

PLEASURE COMES FROM THE WHOLE BODY

The first kisses of adolescence, lips together . . . Then more serious kissing where the tongues wrap round each other . . . Tender or sensual, these 'kisses of life' give rise to some wonderful feelings which flow right through one's body. As one Alfred de Musset once wrote: "The only true language in the world is a kiss."

A kiss is often the first intimate contact between two people.

"I was 15 years old," Stephanie recalls. "At school there was a boy roughly the same age as me who had contrived to arrive and leave at exactly the same time. After a short while he started accompanying me back home. I didn't complain.

"One day, in the front porch, he put his arm round me and drew his face against mine so that his mouth touched the corner of my lips. Then slowly and gently, with just the slightest movement of the head, his lips brushed my mouth from one side to the other. I suddenly felt very excited – and happy. Automatically, my lips parted and he slipped his tongue into my mouth. I felt his warm breath. The excitement mounted inside me. I will never forget that first kiss."

This story well illustrates the feelings that are common to all adolescents when their sensuality starts to be aroused. A kiss that is firm, deep and a touch provocative can produce fluid in the vagina and penis, particularly among young people who have had little or no experience of sexual relations. With some young men this can result in ejaculation. Such was the case with Simon.

"I was 17 and madly in love with my neighbour Valerie, a pretty brunette just a year younger than me. I found every possible excuse to meet and speak with her and to touch her hands or her face.
"One day, she agreed to come to the cinema with me. We sat right at the back where there were very few people. I made the most of the dark to cuddle up to Valerie. I ran my fingers over her lips and then, leaning over her, I licked her mouth with my tongue. As it opened, our tongues met. Her saliva had a delicate taste of violets.
"Our mouths were a source of indescribable pleasure. Valerie gasped quietly and I felt her body quiver. At the same time, I could feel my penis growing. Then, suddenly, I came. I have to say that I felt ashamed at this. Happily, Valerie didn't notice anything."

One interesting thing to note in this story is that Simon sensed the taste of violets in Valerie's mouth. It is actually very important that, when you are kissing sensually, there are not any unpleasant odours – tobacco, garlic or onions, for example. A simple remedy to this problem is the use of toothpaste, sweets or chewing gum. However, it must be said that in a passionate relationship some people do prefer the natural taste of their loved one's mouth.

If kissing can give rise to such sensations, it is above all because the mouth, the tongue and the mucous membranes are very rich in nerve corpuscles which pick up impressions and transmit them to the rest of the body. Moreover, the woman's mouth evokes thoughts of the vagina. Both are warm and damp and the introduction of the tongue is symbolic of penetration of the penis.

From the man's point of view, an 'erect' tongue represents the penis in erection. Kissing is therefore an act of possession, just like making love through penetration.

From the first, timid kiss, deeper kissing generally follows, as tongues play with each other and saliva is exchanged. And the emotional charge that these activities carry produces an erotic effect which releases desire.

You will see later on how deep kissing is often part of the prelude to making love and how many couples kiss spontaneously and furiously at the moment of orgasm.

Kinds of kissing

* If either partner keeps the eyes shut while kissing, this indicates the person has a romantic nature and falls easily in love but does not stay very long.
* If your partner keeps the eyes wide open when you kiss him or her, this denotes someone with a sincere and direct character, capable of an attachment for life.
* Those who kiss their partners like a bird pecking, with their lips together, are hiding a sensual and passionate nature.
* Those kissing with the mouth completely shut reveal a less generous personality, while those who kiss with their lips apart and their tongues active have a particularly passionate temperament.

KISSING ACCORDING TO THE KAMA SUTRA

Some pretend that there is no order or fixed time for embracing, kissing, hugging or caressing, but that all these actions must normally occur before two people finally make love. Equally, there are special actions and noises that generally accompany this particular act.

Vatsyayana, the supposed author of the *Kama Sutra*, believes that anything goes if the moment is right. Love has no cares, no order, no time.

With the very first contact, you should behave with moderation, whether kissing or making any other physical approach. Do not overdo it and, equally, vary your actions. However, on subsequent occasions, you can begin to be more generous in your affection, spend more time and combine all the different actions to arouse the emotions of your partner.

Parts of the body to be kissed include the forehead, the eyes, the cheeks, the throat, the chest, the breasts, the lips and the inside of the mouth. Other sensitive parts include the back of the thighs, the arms and the navel.

But Vatsyayana is of the opinion that, while such people kiss in this way through an outburst of love and through local custom, it is not necessarily a habit that everyone would find agreeable to imitate . . .

For the young girl of today, there are three basic types of kissing – the affectionate kiss, the exciting kiss and the moving kiss.

* The **affectionate kiss** is the simple contact of lips with those of your partner. No other action is involved.
* The **exciting kiss**, which is slightly less modest, comes with moving the bottom lip – but not the upper one – as your partner's mouth presses against yours.
* The **moving kiss** involves touching tongues with your lover and shutting your eyes as you hold hands.

Reference is often made to four other types of kiss – the straight kiss, the leaning kiss, the turned kiss and the pressed kiss.

* The **straight kiss** is when the lips of two lovers meet full-on.
* The **leaning kiss** is when you hang your heads towards each other and then kiss.
* The **turned kiss** is when one of the partners turns towards the other and takes hold of the chin and then kisses.
* The **pressed kiss** is when the bottom lips are pressed firmly against each other.

There is also a fifth sort, known as the heavily pressed kiss. This involves taking the bottom lip between two fingers and then, having touched it with the tongue, pressing the lips strongly together.

On this subject, here is an extract from *Kama Sutra*:

As far as kissing is concerned, you can play at what will create the first response from your partner's lips.

If the woman is taken unawares, she will pretend to start crying, push her lover away by clapping her hands, turn her back on him and pick a quarrel by saying: "Just wait till I get my own back."

If it happens a second time, she will appear doubly distressed. And while her lover is not paying attention or is sleeping, she will take his bottom lip and hold it between her teeth in such a way that it cannot escape. Then she will burst out laughing, create plenty of noise, make fun of her partner and dance right round him, saying whatever comes into her head, rolling her eyes and raising her eyebrows.

Such are the games and squabbles involved with kissing. But the same can be associated with rubbing or scratching with the nails or fingers, with biting and nibbling. However, such habits tend only to be common among those with intense passion.

When the man kisses the upper lip of his partner and she in return kisses his lower lip, this is known as the upper-lip kiss.

When one takes the other's two lips between their own, this is called the clenching kiss. But, with women, this is only practised on men without moustaches. And if, with this kiss, one of the lovers touches with their tongue the teeth, the tongue and the palate of the other, one calls this the tongue fight. This is the time to practise, in the same way, pressing one's teeth against the partner's mouth.

Kissing basically falls into one of four categories: gentle, agressive, hard and soft, depending on which part of the body is involved. Different parts of the body demand different types of kisses.

When a woman looks at her lover's face while he is sleeping and kisses him to display her intention or desire, this is called a kiss that stirs up love.

When a woman kisses her lover while he is working or having an argument with her or looking at something else in such a way as to attract his attention, this is a distracting kiss.

When a lover, returning late at night, kisses his mistress while she is asleep in her bed to demonstrate his desire, one refers to this as a waking kiss. Equally, the woman can pretend to be sleeping when her lover comes home so that she can find out his intention and obtain his respect.

When someone kisses the image of the person they love which is reflected in a mirror, in the water or on a wall, this is known as a kiss that shows intention.

When someone kisses a child sitting on their knee or a painting, an image or a figure in the presence of the person they love, one calls this a transferred kiss.

When at night, in the theatre or during a caste meeting, a man passing in front of a woman kisses one of her fingers, if she is standing, or a toe-nail, if she is seated, or when a woman, who is massaging her lover's body, lays her face on his thigh as if she wanted to sleep and in such a way as to arouse his passion and then kisses his thigh or his big toe-nail, this is called a demonstrative kiss.

Vatsyayana, *Kama Sutra*

A TURNING-POINT IN LIFE

Making love for the first time is a turning-point in life, the memory of which everyone guards as a souvenir. The partner's face and body remain engraved on one's mind, as do the place, the circumstances, the emotion felt, the depth of pleasure ... or, maybe, the difficulties encountered.

We would not go so far as to state that the first sexual experience affects all future ones. But it does leave traces which can sometimes influence sexual behaviour.

How many fears must one overcome and how much love must one both give and receive in order that this first experience is not a failure?

It is important to remember that boys and girls do not live in the same way. The male virgin is familiar with his penis, an external organ he can examine and touch. Generally he has already experienced the pleasure of masturbation. He knows that copulation brings no anatomical change whatsoever to his penis and does not have to be concerned – as is the case with young girls – about the penetration of another sexual organ into his body.

But he does worry about his inexperience and is afraid of not knowing how to 'set about it' or that his partner might laugh at him. And what about the boy, over eighteen and still a virgin, who has a complex about it? This only increases his shyness in front of girls and his embarrassment in front of his friends who have themselves already taken the plunge and freely boast about it.

It is important that men know certain simple and reassuring facts about the female psychology, such as:

* The presence of the hymen, which is not the impenetrable barrier some novices in love believe it to be.
* The need for lubrication of the vagina, which is self-producing all the time the desire exists.
* The capacity of the vagina to accept an erect penis, whatever its size.

Young men must also be aware that their partners need, at that special moment, to hear tender words, be caressed gently and to be fully prepared for this initiation into love-making. However burning the desire, men must not get carried away into acting violently or too rapidly, which could otherwise wound their partners both psychologically and physically.

If, as has already been said, a girl does not live the first experience in the same way as a boy, this is essentially due to the fact that the loss of one's virginity is too often referred to as a painful exercise, to which one is resigned to submit. Even today, some

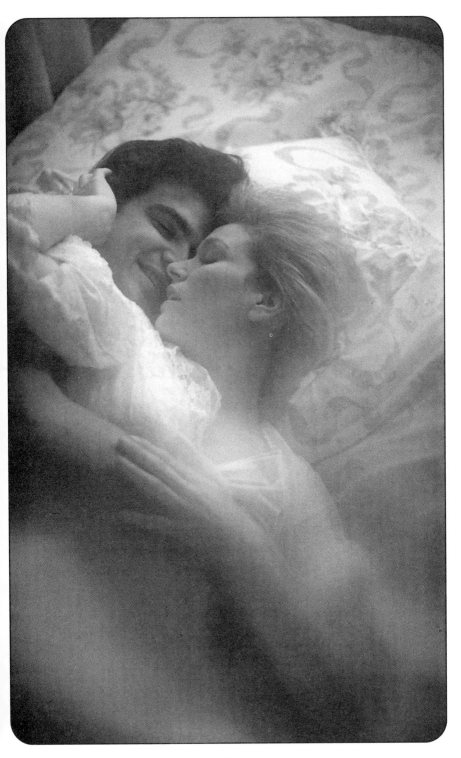

literature, cinema and sometimes families themselves carry this kind of prejudice.

To avoid such misleading ideas, it is important to know one's own body (*see page 16*) – and not just those sexual organs you can see, but also those inside that remain invisible.

For example, the muscles in the vulva, which contract through fear of the first experience, make the penetration of the penis into the vagina more difficult.

Equally important to consider are the characteristics of the hymen, the thin elastic membrane which partly closes the vagina. Pierced in the middle by a small opening which allows for the discharge during periods, this membrane is broken during the first sexual intercourse as the penis enters the vagina. This laceration is not necessarily painful or followed by bleeding.

The lack of the hymen is, however, no proof whatsoever that a girl has lost her virginity. It could well have been broken during some strenuous physical exercise, such as horse-riding, ballet dancing or cycling.

To these fears one must also add that of becoming pregnant, despite the fact that some girls are persuaded – wrongly, of course – that there is absolutely no risk of this happening the first time they make love.

Those who already take the pill run no risk of this kind. Others must count on the sense of responsibility of their partner, whose only available contraceptive will be the condom.

Thus a young couple decide to put their shared feelings of love and a desire to belong totally to each other to the test and make love for the first time.

Privacy is essential, whether inside or outdoors. Kissing and caressing will have excited the man to the point of erection, while for the woman the vagina will now be sufficiently lubricated to enable the penetration and free movement of the penis.

The woman lays down on her back, with a cushion under her bottom. She bends her knees and opens her thighs. The man lays on top of her and enters her in this position, which not only exposes the vagina but also stretches the hymen, thus making it easier to break.

When this happens, in about two-thirds of the cases bleeding will occur to a lesser or greater extent. The couple should not be worried by this or the brief pain that the woman will then experience.

The in-and-out movement of the penis, in a rhythm at first slow and then accelerating, will eventually cause ejaculation. The time this takes will depend on the individual. The sperm will shoot out into the vagina in fits and starts. This is the male orgasm.

The female orgasm does not necessarily happen at the same moment. And it can be that the woman is not even conscious of it when she experiences sexual intercourse for the first time. But even if she does not reach a state of orgasm this time, she will still undergo a very different and much stronger pleasure than that felt when kissing and caressing.

This, in very simple terms, is what happens when a man and a woman make love successfully for the first time. Let us now look at what else can sometimes occur in this situation.

If the man is in a very anxious state, he can lose his erection and therefore will not be able to penetrate the vagina. If this happens, a little time spent relaxing and sharing affection will help him recover his erection.

Another problem, again caused by worry, can be that the woman's vaginal muscles contract to the point where penetration becomes impossible. Here again, relaxation and some tenderness are recommended before trying again.

More difficult is the case where the erect penis does not manage to break through the hymen, possibly because it is too resistant or not perforated. Here the only solution to the problem is a medical one and it will be necessary to delay that first experience until all the conditions are favourable.

SOME TESTIMONIES

Two people here recall their first sexual experience, beginning with a woman.

Gaye (age 30)

"I was 18, the same age as Edward. When we weren't studying, we spent all our free time together. We were constantly making plans for the future. Yes, we were going to get married as soon as we started to earn a living. It was the real thing. More and more we needed to be near each other, to touch each other, to kiss each other. Love was certainly burning inside both of us.

"One day, Edward asked me if I would like to do it. Yes, I said, I would. To tell you the truth, I had been dreaming of nothing else. His parents had a flat above a hairdressing salon they managed, which they never left all day. This meant we could use his bedroom without being disturbed.

"The windows were shut and the curtains drawn. We were standing face to face in front of the bed which I hardly dared to look at. Gently and discreetly, Edward took off my coat, unbuttoned my blouse and started stroking my breasts with one hand while he took off my skirt with the other. Soon I stood naked in the semi-darkness of the room.

"Edward then took me in his arms and laid me gently on the bed. I shut my eyes, worried stiff with anxiety about what was going to happen. He laid down naked beside me and began stroking me all over, at the same time whispering sweet words of love. I felt afraid but at the same time wanted him to take me. I felt the weight of his body on mine and his hard penis against my vagina. Instinctively I opened my thighs and, with a single thrust, he went right inside me. I felt a very sharp, but brief, pain like burning. I cried out. Edward stopped inside me and for a while didn't move.

"I felt no more pain and the penis of the man I loved in my stomach began to give me a feeling of well-being, of fullness. He started to move up and down very slowly. My fear had gone. The feeling of pleasure I experienced was certainly not what I had imagined it would be. It filled my whole body. Then suddenly Edward speeded up and, after a few moments, he fell on top of me groaning. I felt an enormous warmth in my stomach.

"We stayed like that for what seemed an eternity. My head was in a complete spin.

"When Edward finally withdrew, I saw that I had been bleeding. But very little, less than I had feared. I honestly thought at the time that I had really haemorrhaged.

"That is how I remember my first time. I should add that for me the real pleasure and final orgasm only came after two or three times of making love."

Ralph

"I was twenty years old, still a virgin and proud to be so. I should add that girls frightened me to the point where I would run away from them while at the same time dreaming of holding them in my arms. All the same I did finally manage it, although I must admit completely by chance.

"Pamela was eighteen and the god-daughter of my step-father (my mother was widowed and remarried when I was sixteen) when she came to spend three weeks holiday with us in the country. We had a good time together, walking in the forest and swimming in the nearby river. I felt really at ease with her. She was high-spirited and very natural.

"It was in fact Pamela who very quickly made the first move when she asked me to kiss her. How delightful that was! We made the most of all future opportunities to kiss and caress.

"Finally, one night, I decided to go into her bedroom. I confessed to her that I had no experience and she replied that for her too it would be the first time. I fancied her so much that I already had an erection. That worried me since I was afraid she would think I was too clumsy. It was even worse than that! When I wanted to enter her, my penis had gone all soft.

"I was horrified and ashamed. But Pamela got hold of my penis to help me recover my virility and gradually it hardened up again. In the meantime I was conjuring up all sorts of fantasies to get myself excited. Finally it worked.

"For some unexpected reason to do with the family, she had to leave the following day. I didn't dare start with another girl. However, this first experience has, despite the setback I suffered, helped me understand two important points. Firstly, I had given pleasure to a pretty and interesting young girl. So why not others like her? Secondly, I had gained a lot more pleasure than through my customary masturbations.

"These observations eventually encouraged me to try my luck with a friend of my sister. This time there was no problem. My real sex life was on the right track and I haven't looked back since."

The first time?

It is not always the case that both the man and the woman are experiencing sex for the first time. One or other of them could already have had intercourse. So does this guarantee a successful initiation for the other party?

Previous generations have thought so and some went as far as to favour the sexual initiation of a young man by an older woman who could teach him the finer points of making love, as well as alleviating his fears and removing his clumsiness.

Apparently young women were not allowed quite the same freedom, since their virginity was considered a treasure – an asset exclusively reserved for the married man.

Today, young people meet, fall in love and very often make love before getting married. It is becoming increasingly rare for a man to arrive at his wedding night a virgin. But a woman's virginity continues to carry a certain value. Following an enquiry by one Dr David Elia, 27 per cent of men considered the woman's virginity fundamental, 35 per cent thought it was important but not that much and 16 per cent said that it had no importance at all.

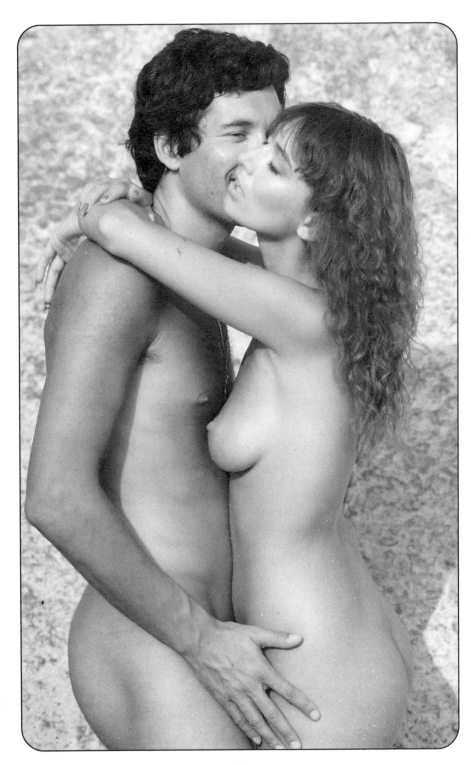

2

THE KNOW-HOW OF LOVE

*From the erotic awakening
to the sexual awareness –
the foundation of a couple's happiness*

THE PRELUDE: BODY TALK

It is the amorous session that precedes sexual intercourse – involving kissing, embracing, touching, whispering and a thousand and one caresses – which stirs up desire and opens the doors of pleasure.

A quote from a doctor, who specialises in sexuality is significant. "In very simple terms, sexuality passes through four successive stages during a session of love-making: seduction, caressing and kissing, undressing and finally the search for orgasm."

Two of these stages, caressing and kissing and then undressing, form part of the foreplay. How this is carried out will depend on the individual's sensuality, also his or her age and the quality of the emotional links with the other person involved.

The degree of sensuality, which is attributed to everyone who enjoys the pleasures of the senses, varies from individual to individual, whether male or female. However, sensuality is in everyone, even if it is not immediately evident or is in some way inhibited by prejudice or an over-strict education.

It is a 'Sleeping Beauty' which must be awoken from the moment of those first adolescent contacts in order to blossom in adults and continue throughout life, even into old age. And the art of arousing the senses and learning to satisfy their requirements, which is essential for the happiness and harmony of any couple, must come over a period of time.

The preliminaries to sex involve the sharing of intimate gestures which will produce sensual feelings and prepare the two bodies for that final, successful union.

A couple who love each other will always know how to find the time for this foreplay, even if it sometimes happens that by chance they are caught on the hop or, through some particular circumstance, are forced to improvise.

Foreplay is, without doubt, an essential element of a loving and erotic relationship. We have already pointed out that everyone lives the experience according to their age. While the very young are not always capable of controlling their enthusiasm and end up reaching a state of orgasm too quickly, more mature lovers will benefit from their joint experiences.

The quality of the emotional link between partners plays its part equally in this preliminary session before love-making. Through love one knows instinctively what will satisfy and, equally, what could upset one's partner. True love carries such an understanding of each other that all one's shared desires are met.

How much time should one devote to foreplay?

It is obviously impossible to give a specific answer as to the exact period, since this is such a personal affair. We can only give rough guidelines from statistics published in a recent report on the sexual behaviour of Europeans.

According to those questioned in the report, foreplay lasted as follows: less than 5 minutes – 16 per cent; 5-9 minutes – 27 per cent; 15-17 minutes – 9 per cent; 20-29 minutes – 6 per cent; and around 30 minutes – 3 per cent.

To elaborate on this, take the example of a couple – Mary and William – who are 29 and 33 respectively and have been married for eight years. This is what happens in their foreplay – or, more accurately, one typical occasion, since it is certainly not a standard ritual with established rules, but a series of sensual gestures which can vary according to the moment and, of course, the imagination.

Starting with deep, full-mouth kissing, with their tongues intertwining passionately, William then slides his lips down Mary's neck as he gently nibbles at her ear. He kneels down behind her, puts his hands on her breasts and gently fingers her nipples, which swell up and harden. Their caresses become more specific: pinching the nipples, tickling tongues, breathing into each other's mouths. Mary begins to feel hot flushes in her lower abdomen, her thighs start throbbing with excitement and her vagina moistens in preparation to receive her husband's penis.

Now William explores the rest of her body with his mouth, while he puts his hand on her Mount of Venus. Then he pushes open the outer lips and searches for the button of the clitoris, which he begins to masturbate excitedly.

Mary is overcome with pleasure, while at the same time arousing her partner by stroking his penis before taking it firmly in her hand.

Just for a moment, they interrupt these sensual exchanges to change position. Mary lays on her side to give William the chance to look at and stroke her back. He runs his fingernails down the length of her spine, then works his finger into the clamminess of her bottom. This creates the most sensual reactions in Mary who, for her part, increases her partner's excitment by passionately kissing his body from top to toe, dwelling on the most sensitive spots such as the inside of the thighs, the penis, the navel, the nipples and the armpits.

Thanks to such erotic play, where love is able to express itself imaginatively and freely, each can experience uninhibited pleasure right up to the marvellous moment where William's urge to enter Mary – or her's to accept him – takes over with such force that the lovers' bodies become as one to reach the ultimate climax of pleasure.

Research by sexologists during the Fifties and Sixties revealed that the sexual reactions of women were slower than those of men and that they therefore needed foreplay – and particularly caressing – to prepare them for the moment of orgasm. Even if this is not always the case for men, they certainly enjoy this as much as their partner.

Love-making normally takes place in the privacy of a bedroom. But there are other places equally intimate and provocative – such as in front of an open fire or on the couch. And, weather permitting, some like to make love outside in some discreet corner out of sight.

According to a nationwide opinion poll in 1985, 57 per cent of those questioned said they made love in a car, while 55 per cent admitted having sex in the open air. So this is certainly not something that is confined to the bedroom!

Whatever the time or the place, foreplay generally starts with serious kissing. While the tongues play, the hands join in, undoing the clothes and sliding over the bare skin, pausing when they reach the sensitive spots – the nape of the neck, the rim of the ears, the breasts. Soon the mouth takes over from the hands, sucking and licking the erogenous zones.

The hands are busy stripping the body of clothes, the tips of the fingers following the contours of the belly button and moving down as far as the sexual organ, stroking it lightly at first, then more seriously. Reciprocal masturbation and the brushing of the cheek on the genital organs creates an excitement so intense that the man risks ejaculating.

Two people experimenting must learn how to recognise the moment where they have to stop the caressing to lower the sexual tension. If the partners are novices in love-making, the man should be conscious of his own reactions and not wait till the point of no return – that of ejaculating – to make that subtle transfer from foreplay to the final act of making love.

It can happen that the woman experiences one or even several orgasms during foreplay. This should not hinder her from further enjoyment when her partner enters her. In effect, the woman has the advantage of being able to experience a number of orgasms in the course of foreplay and the sexual act, while the man, once he has ejaculated, cannot make love again immediately.

The celebrated American sexologists Dr William Masters and Virginia Johnson discovered that for men three ejaculations in one hour represented a real feat, while for women five or six orgasms in the same period of time were quite possible. This is explained by the differences of physiological characteristics between the sexes *(see Orgasm page 62).*

The temperament of each individual plays a part in the preliminaries of love-play, whether it is that the two partners have the same tastes for a certain kind of caressing or whether they differ and this conflict of tastes is in itself a source of excitement.

SOME TESTIMONIES

Judith

"I am a young romantic and our bedroom reflects my tastes. I feel really comfortable in it, particularly when my husband comes up to caress me before making love. While I am soft and gentle, with the surrounding decor of muslin curtains, of precious opals, of trees of faraway islands, I only gain pleasure in foreplay when Bruce is agressive. I love it when he pushes me around a little, taps and even pinches me. In contrast, I caress him softly and tenderly... We make the foreplay last as long as possible, interrupting our love-play with passive moments where we simply lie wrapped together embracing each other."

Audrey

"We get undressed together and, in the nude, we stand and passionately embrace each other. Then Edmund touches my breasts, tickles the nipples and kisses them. His hands then explore the whole of my body until his fingers sink into my vagina... I listen to his heaving breath. I take his penis and I rub it against me. We remain standing. This is how the foreplay excites us most."

Mary

"For me there is a definite pattern to our caressing. Terry starts with my breasts, then moves down to the lips of my vulva and then my clitoris. His mouth and his fingers create such an excitement, which increases by the second. When I am on the edge of an orgasm, I tear myself away from his caresses and it is my turn to stimulate every square inch of his body, from the roots of his hair to the tips of his toes. This is our great session of foreplay to which we each surrender when we have the time."

Rose
"John is truly the man in my life. He contributes so much to my happiness through his tenderness, his attentions and his constant concern for my well-being. He loves my body above all and, when we are together, he describes it to me in passionate terms, right down to the smallest detail. When we go to bed in the evening, he asks me to get undressed like a striptease artist. With very slow and deliberate movements, I take off my blouse, lifting my arms high in the air to show him my armpits with their light gold covering of hair. Then I remove my bra and caress my breasts. After that, I let my skirt slip down to the floor as I wiggle my hips, revealing my small panties and suspender belt. I undo my stockings and roll each one slowly down to the bottom of my leg. All this time John, who is stretched out on the bed, watches my performance with eyes glued. This is one type of foreplay that excites me as much as it does him."

Alison
"Steve and I have been married for eight years, during which time he has given me all the sexual satisfaction any woman could want. But in order to get going, he first has to look at pictures of nudes in girly magazines. He likes me to stretch out alongside him while he flicks through the pages and he takes my hand and puts it on his penis. I can feel it throbbing and then swelling. Once he has a good erection, he throws the magazine to one side and starts to caress me all over, sometimes gently and sometimes more firmly. This makes me so excited I could explode. I am a happy woman, both emotionally and sensually, but to me this need of Simon to look at nude pin-ups before making love does seem rather degrading – for him as well as for me. I did speak to him about it and he explained that it was a habit that went back to his adolescence and to have integrated that into our sex life appeared to him one futher link between us."

Women and men
As we have already mentioned, women are slower in getting excited than men, for whom the pleasure in foreplay is limited to a few caresses, especially among those under fifty.

Having got past this age, the build-up tends to last longer, which does not generally bring any protest from the woman since she thus benefits from a longer exchange of caresses. However that may be, even if the man is satisfied with only a brief foreplay, he does nonetheless gain pleasure from provoking and watching that of his partner.

Arnold (age 30)
"My wife only has to touch my penis for me to get an erection. But I know that Angela is not ready to make love so quickly. At the start of our marriage, I hadn't understood that. I was following my desires, persuaded that she wanted the same. When I found out, some time later, that she wasn't reaching the climax or enjoying an orgasm, I began asking myself questions. I even discussed the matter with a medical friend of mine. He explained the female physiology and psychology to me and particularly the body's need to prepare for penetration. Ever since then our sex life has changed for the better and I am now really happy to see the excitement building up on Angela's face."

Albert (age 58)
"Even six or eight years ago I was getting an erection as soon as Emily stimulated my penis. A few seconds were enough. Now it takes several minutes of touching and stroking with the hands and cheek for my friend to reach a satisfactory hardness. Emily is quite happy to join in the playing, because I do the same for her. For although having passed her menopause, her sexuality is still very much alive, thanks to a hormone treatment she has been undergoing for the last ten years. I read somewhere that couples devote less and less time to the preliminaries as they grow older. In my opinion, this is not true. One can be sexually aroused even when one reaches what they call 'old age'. My wife and I can prove it!"

THE SENSUAL MESSAGE: RELAXATION AND AROUSAL

Hands are alive. They move about as you please. Thanks to the multiple nerve endings in them, they have a marvellous power of sensitivity and they play a major role in your overall sensuality.

Whether your caresses are delicate or firm, when massaging arouses the passion the real pleasure comes from the tips of your fingers. So learn some of the simple techniques to relax the body and prepare it for love-making.

For an effective erotic massage, you must take your time. Make the most of a long, quiet evening or even a weekend. Create an ambiance that is agreeable, soft and intimate: subdued lighting, gentle music, perfumed candles, a bed or mattress on the floor.

Start off by taking a shower or bath together. Wash every part of each other's body and then dry each other all over using soft towels.

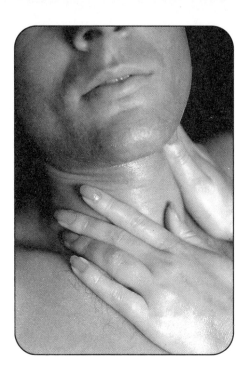

Some people like to be dried 'Indian style', that is to say with the naked hand. Each rubs the other's body until the skin is dry. This method of drying can often be very exciting.

Now you are ready for the massage. You are both naked. One of you is going to play the active role, the other the passive role. You can reverse the roles the second time round.

To simplify the explanation of the technique, we have taken one particular couple – Tina and Francis – as an example. They have been practising sensual massaging for more than three years and have derived enormous benefit, as much from the relaxation it produces as from the sexual pleasure it provides.

Tina starts by taking the active role. She coats her hands with a perfumed oil, while Francis stretches out on his back, with his head on the floor, his arms by his side and his knees bent, with his feet pressing firmly against the side of the couch.

When he is in position, Tina kneels down behind his head and, with her fingers and the palms of her hand, she lightly massages his chest from bottom to top, that is to say from his stomach up towards his shoulders. Francis breathes in deeply when her hands are around his plexus and then breathes out slowly as she moves up to his shoulders. This exercise, which lasts about five minutes, creates a feeling of relaxation and well-being. And this feeling mounts with the following exercise:

Tina places her right hand close to Francis' stomach and her left hand close to his chest without either of them touching his body. He in turn breathes in deeply through his chest and then his stomach so that, as each expands, it touches Tina's hands. He then breathes out slowly. This is repeated eight times.

After this, Tina puts her hands on either side of Francis' neck and works her fingers around it, vigorously massaging the nape with her thumbs. She repeats this five or six times, while he continues to breathe in and out. A combination of breathing and massage greatly assists in the process of relaxation.

Next, Francis sits with his legs doubled up and his hands on his thighs. Tina kneels behind him and massages his scalp with her fingertips, before stroking his hair and then working down on to his shoulders, his back and his hips, all the time with a highly sensual touch.

Then the two of them kneel in front of each other as Tina runs her lips slowly over Francis' face and chest. She keeps this up for several minutes before sliding her hands and mouth over his whole body, pausing over the most sensitive spots, such as the nipples, the inside of the thighs and even the genital parts.

When the excitement reaches its peak, she stops and the two then lie down side by side for several moments, with their eyes closed, breathing deeply and keeping contact by holding hands.

For the next stage, Francis lies flat on his stomach and Tina sits astride him and massages his back. She then lies full length on top of him and stays there for two or three minutes.

So the massage, which fulfils the dual role of relaxation and excitement, is over. And it is now the turn of the passive partner to adopt the active role and give to the other the same sensations that he or she has just experienced.

THE MOST INTIMATE LOVE-MAKING

There is one kind of love-making, both tender and daring, which some people practise that involves contact betwen the mouth and the genital organs. This is known as oral sex. A source of infinite pleasure, it is yet another variation on the erotic games played by couples who are already united by a deep and meaningful relationship. Oral stimulation of the penis is known as fellatio and that of the vagina cunnilingus.

These practices date back to the mists of time and have been described by some of the great writers of erotic literature – Vatsyayana, Sade, Verlaine and Henry Miller.

But is this form of love-making really obscene, as some people would have us believe? Our reply is that between two people who love each other and want to be completely fulfilled in their sexual relationship, such practices undertaken in the strictest intimacy cannot possibly be considered obscene.

Those with a strict upbringing, based on traditional prejudices, have doubtless been taught to consider the sexual organs as 'dirty' and, consequently, their contact with the mouth as unclean. This idea is fundamentally false, since the penis and vagina receive the same hygienic care as the rest of the body. And if the words 'dirty' and 'unclean' are taken in the moral sense, then this is a grave mistake, even the denial of sexuality through the refusal of the sexual organs.

Quite clearly, each individual's sensibility plays a part here and must be respected. Fellatio and cunnilingus are not part of the love-making one should demand from the first encounter. One must already have a perfect understanding with one's partner, of their body, of their likes and dislikes, just as much as one's own, before embarking on oral sex.

Of course, this can be an important part of foreplay without being the very first act. It can also be practised in the course of copulation, through sexual play or to revive a failing erection.

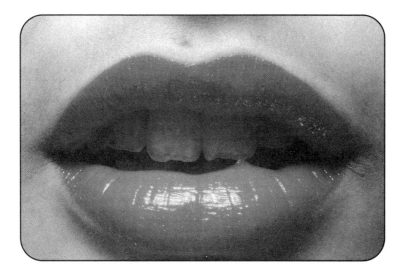

FELLATIO

The woman takes her partner's penis in her mouth. She nibbles it and sucks it, licking the gland and moving her lips up and down the penis. Some women remain reticent about this kind of lovemaking. They feel sick at the feeling of a penis penetrating their throat and find the smell and taste unpleasant. And if the sperm is ejected into their mouth, they consider this disgusting.

Such feelings must be made known to one's partner, who on no account should try to impose his desire for fellatio. Instead the couple should try other things, such as limiting oral activity to the gland or withdrawing the penis from the mouth at the moment of ejaculation.

And while the woman performs fellatio on her partner, he in turn should stimulate her in such a way as to maximize her excitement.

CUNNILINGUS

This involves the man kissing his partner's vulva, the inner and outer lips and the clitoris with his mouth and tongue. The tongue then penetrates the vagina like a miniature penis. All the while, he inhales the exciting smell of the female sexual parts.

It is rare for women not to be lifted to the height of pleasure when their partner performs cunnilingus.

IN WHAT POSITIONS SHOULD ONE PRACTISE ORAL SEX?

To perform fellatio, the man can be stretched out on his back with the woman between his open thighs. She can also turn her back and sit astride him, thus presenting her backside to her partner. If he is sitting, she can kneel between his legs. Even if he is standing up, she can do the same.

To receive cunnilingus, the woman can adopt any position that enables her to expose her vulva – stretched out with thighs open, knees bent and bust slightly raised with some cushions underneath; or with her legs resting on her partner's shoulders, her vagina within reach of his mouth.

And there is, of course, the well-known position known as 'soixante-neuf' (69), where the man and woman lie one on top of each other, head to foot and with legs apart, so that each can practise oral sex on the other at the same time.

AN INTIMATE SECRET

Those who practise oral sex rarely admit to doing so – whether through discretion or through fear of being criticised or judged to be lewd. Thus this great feast of sensuality remains the couples' intimate secret.

From information gleaned through confidential interviews and discussion, sexologists believe that the taboos surrounding this area of love-making are beginning to disappear and that the numbers of people who indulge in oral sex between the age of twenty-five and forty-five are growing.

One fairly recent European survey included the following statistics: of the 100,000 women interviewed, 8 per cent confirmed that their husband or lover practised cunnilingus, while 80 per cent regularly practised fellatio.

One can draw the conclusion from this survey that men are fondled more than women when it comes to oral sex. Since more than ten years has elapsed since the report was made, one can only hope that, with the continual change in attitudes to morality and the growth in sexual equality, the woman's situation has improved at the same time.

SOME TESTIMONIES

Lydia (age 31)
"I have never dared ask my husband to perform cunnilingus. I am afraid that he will not like the smell of my vagina and that the thought of putting his mouth there will revolt him."

Anika (age 27)
"My husband practised cunnilingus on several occasions. I find the word somewhat crude and prefer to use the term 'to lick my vagina'. I came so strongly each time and had such violent orgasms that I was afraid that I would no longer gain pleasure from other things. So we have stopped."

Jane (age 33)
"In ten years of living together and enjoying a good sexual relationship, my husband has never practised cunnilingus, although he frequently asks me to perform fellatio on him. I dream about experiencing the pleasure I have never known. But my discretion prevents me from asking for it."

Angela (age 29)
"We regularly practise oral sex. I love to have Carl's penis in my mouth. What I didn't appreciate at all was the taste of the sperm when he ejaculated. I had to tell him as much. Now he withdraws his penis from my mouth just before he comes. He is a true husband and a marvellous lover."

Victor (age 40)

"My wife refuses to perform fellatio on me. She finds the whole idea 'dirty'. We have been married for twelve years now and my desire for this type of sex is so strong that I am beginning to wonder whether I shouldn't look for it elsewhere."

Graham (age 38)

"When Mel takes my penis in her mouth and starts to suck it, I get such wonderful sensations all over. I tell her about them and express my pleasure with groans of delight. When I reach orgasm, she comes too."

THE ABSOLUTE PLEASURE

ORGASM . . . DYING OF PLEASURE

The highest point of sexual pleasure is accompanied by strong, sometimes even violent, sensations which can lead up to temporary loss of consciousness. Orgasm is often also called the 'little death'. But, quite obviously, there is absolutely nothing to fear from these totally pleasurable experiences.

We know that orgasm is brought about in several ways: through masturbation, through fondling particularly sensitive parts of the body, which vary from person to person, and through coitus.

Whatever its cause, orgasm does in principle bring the same pleasure. We say 'in principle', because if auto-eroticism does create powerful feelings, one's sexual life cannot be easily contained. In our opinion, sex is only truly fulfilling between two people, with all their bodily characteristics – the texture of the skin, the hair, the body odour and so on.

Let us look now at what a couple can experience at the moment of orgasm.

With certain exceptions, which we will examine later, for the man, orgasm accompanies ejaculation. With it, he experiences intense delight. But men in general do not speak openly about their orgasms. They do not know how – or are not willing – to describe them. So testimonies about this part of love-making are rare. Those that we do have tend to come from women who have observed their partners at the time, such as:

"His face winced as if he was suffering."

"He rolled his eyes and gritted his teeth."
"He let out several weak groans."
"His body convulsed all over."

As far as women are concerned, they describe their orgasms in often dreamlike terms – 'sinking in an ocean of desire', 'exploding like a firework', 'hearing heavenly choirs' and 'being in another world'.

Angela, who is twenty-four, expresses her feelings as follows: "I float in the clouds, high up in the sky; my body is weightless; streaks of colour pass under my closed eyelids."

And for Sophie, who is thirty-seven: "My body bursts into a thousand pieces; I have fireworks in my head; I feel immortal."

And thirty-two-year-old Joyce: "Apparently when I reach my orgasm I cry out as if I was in great pain. My husband told me this. I have no idea, since at that moment I am completely unconscious."

In the words of Alex, who is thirty: "When I started having a sexual relationship with Sandra, I was startled by the violence of her orgasms. Her whole body trembled and she was quite incoherent, as if in a state of delirium. Then, after a few seconds, her body stopped moving and she slept. Her face was pale and totally drained. We have now been married four years and still she reacts in the same way. But it doesn't stop her from being perfectly fresh and alert when she emerges from this sleep."

Another testimony, this time from thirty-one-year-old Ronald, does call for comment. "At the moment of orgasm, my wife emits a lot of colourless and odourless fluid. It's a sort of ejaculation."

This may be rare, but it exists all the same. Through analysis of this female fluid, it has been established that its composition does relate to the male's prostatic fluid.

When reading the descriptions of the explosive female orgasm and the more measured male orgasm, one is led to wonder whether men and women feel the same pleasure. Because, if everyone experienced their own pleasure, we would not know how to confirm whether it was identical or not.

Female sexuality is more complex than the male variety. In order to blossom out erotically, women need a climate of tenderness, while men freely display in their sexuality their instinct for power and domination – even aggression.

It is the virility opposed to the femininity – virility finding self-expression in possession in contrast to the woman's desire to be loved passionately.

As Dr Gilbert Tordjman and Dr Charles Gelman wrote in *The Man & His Pleasure:* "Masculine and feminine pleasure evolve in a context emotionally different . . ." And to quote an enquiry in the magazine *Marie-Claire:* "68 per cent of women give priority to the tenderness in their love life, 8 per cent to the sexual act and 38 per cent would be able to dispense completely with sexual intercourse if they could bathe in a climate of love and understanding."

We said that the woman's sexuality was complex. We have seen that her psycho-emotional responses are more subtle than those of the man. Such complexity exists equally in the physiology of the woman and in her sexual reactions. She responds more slowly to stimulation (it takes a minimum of ten minutes for the woman to pass from the relaxed state to that of orgasm) and is capable of having several successive orgasms and of achieving them by different routes.

This last point is particularly important. It had, for a long time, been believed that the woman only reaches orgasm through vaginal penetration. The work of Dr William Masters and Virginia Johnson in the Sixties provided evidence that it was the stimulation of the clitoris – be it through masturbation or, during intercourse, the rubbing of the penis – that caused orgasm: this is clitoral orgasm, which is experienced by most women.

Is this to say that vaginal orgasm does not in fact exist? While some admit to feeling nothing in their vagina, about 30 per cent do reach orgasm through vaginal intromission.

As Masters and Johnson wrote in their book *Human Sexual Response:* "There is only one sort of orgasm resulting from effective sexual stimulation, the vagina and clitoris reacting according to constant physiological patterns. This is why orgasms, whether vaginal or clitoral, do not constitute separate biological entities."

For Dr Gilbert Tordjman in *The Woman & Her Pleasure:* "The distinction of the two orgasms, the one vaginal and the other clitoral, responds to a subjective, emotional reality . . ." The assertion of Dr Tordjman is corroborated by clinical observations: those women capable of achieving both types of orgasm describe the feelings brought on by the stimulation of the clitoris as "immediate, exacerbated, punctual", while the vaginal orgasm "calls in the partner's personality and a relational dimension".

Simultaneous orgasm

For many couples, completely successful sexual intercourse must finish with simultaneous orgasm, the man and the woman both coming at the same moment.

According to a recent survey, 56 per cent of men and 40 per cent of women achieve orgasm at the same time, the man coming first in 40 per cent of the cases. This is explained on the one hand by the fact that, when a man gets very excited, he can lose control of his ejaculation and on the other hand by the woman's physiology itself – slower to be stirred up sexually and multi-orgasmic.

This desire for simultaneous orgasm is, however, the source of much delusion. The woman feigns orgasm just to satisfy her husband and sometimes also to reassure him, since some men consider it proof of their egoism if they come before their partner. But the important thing is not the simultaneousness of the orgasm, but the orgasm itself.

It is worth noting here a comment from Dr Gilbert Tordjman: "The simultaneousness of the two orgasms – male and female – is not a criterion either for happiness or for satisfaction."

WHAT HAPPENS IN THE WOMAN'S BODY FROM FOREPLAY TO ORGASM

From the build-up of pleasure provoked by sexual stimulation right up to the explosive moment of orgasm, the woman's body experiences some important changes.

Let us go back to the anatomy of the vagina in terms solely of its function as a sexual organ and see how it reacts, from the moment when the woman starts to feel excited right up to the final outcome – orgasm.

Vaginal lubrication

The first reaction to sexual stimulation, whatever form it takes, is vaginal lubrication. We have already seen how the Bartholin glands, concealed inside the thick outer lips near the anus, lubricate the vagina when the desire starts and during the sexual act.

Moreover, the walls of the vagina secrete a kind of 'sweat', some droplets, whose production grows under the effect of such excitement. At the same time the walls of the vagina, which are naturally stuck together, separate. The vaginal passage thus prepares itself in a voluntary and reflex action for the penetration of the penis.

The outer and inner lips

The outer and inner lips open up and swell and the vaginal passage lengthens and swells out along its upper two-thirds. From its initial length of eight or nine centimetres, the vagina reaches eleven or twelve centimetres. The clitoris also lengthens and hardens. We are now in what is known as the 'excitement phase', which was well studied by Masters and Johnson.

In their research, they also described the physiological changes in the vagina in the course of the following phase, known as 'the plateau'. The sexual tension has risen. In its turn, the last third of the vagina, the part nearest to the vaginal opening, also changes. It produces a rush of blood in the veins, thus provoking a congestion of the vaginal walls and reducing the passage by about a third. The inner lips are swollen with blood and there is a further slight increase in the length and width of the other two-thirds of the vagina. The woman is ready to accept the penis, whose girating movements will intensify her sexual excitement even more.

For the woman, this 'plateau phase' normally lasts about ten minutes, while for the man it is on average only around three minutes.

This is followed by the 'orgasmic phase'. The sexual tension is at its height. Orgasm is going to take place and proceed in three stages.

The very first feeling of orgasm in the woman will give her the impression that everything has stopped. That only lasts an instant, immediately followed by a feeling of intense pleasure which starts at the clitoris and then radiates through the whole area of the pelvis.

That is the first stage.

Breathing and heartbeats accelerate

There are some important changes that occur in the woman's body immediately after this first stage. The chest muscles tighten and the breathing, normally ten to fourteen breaths per minute, climbs to forty. The heart accelerates, too, sometimes up to a hundred and eighty beats per minute.

The part of the vagina nearest the opening contracts and then expands repeatedly. The breasts become congested with blood and expand. The nipples harden and the areoles fold as they contract. And red flushes appear on the top of the bust and the neck.

The whole body is filled with warmth

In the second stage, which follows immediately, the sensations spread over the whole body and this is accompanied by a warmth that prompts a wave of sensual delight.

This leads into the start of the third stage, when the woman feels the inner part of her vagina contracting. Almost immediately this is followed by throbbings, strongest in the pelvis but which spread to every part of the body. For its part, the uterus contracts rhythmically at intervals of around eight-tenths of a second.

Masters and Johnson were able to measure the contractions with the help of probes inserted in the uterus itself. They were thus able to establish a scale of intensity for the orgasm. Three to four contractions corresponded to a mild orgasm, five to eight contractions to an average orgasm and eight to twelve contractions to an extreme orgasm.

Thus successive waves of pleasure overwhelm the woman. But even if orgasm follows certain physiological patterns, it is none the less very individual and different for each person.

A woman's orgasm is very short, lasting between three and fifteen seconds.

The sexual tension eases

After orgasm, the sexual tension drops. This is the moment when the woman feels really good, the time of complete relaxation. It is known as the 'resolution phase'.

The body relaxes and there are some physiological changes. The congestion in the pelvis disappears quickly and the lower part of the vagina, which had contracted, opens up again. As a result, the vaginal passage expands. The upper part of the vagina (the internal section enlarged by the excitement) returns to its original size. And the vaginal mucous membrane, which turned violet under the effects of the sexual tension, gradually recovers its normal colour. This takes between ten and fifteen minutes.

The breasts deflate and the red flushes on the bust and the neck disappear. The congestion of the inner lips resorbs. And, in most cases, the vaginal lubrication stops, although it has been known for this to continue, indicating a revival of sexual tension.

WHAT HAPPENS IN THE MAN'S BODY FROM FOREPLAY TO ORGASM

If, for women, the physiological changes occur essentially in the vagina, then for men this takes place in the penis – but also the scrotum, the testicles and the breasts.

We have already described the male's sexual anatomy *(see Chapter 1)*. We must return there to study the reactions of the sexual organs during both foreplay and coitus.

The penis

We will begin with the penis, whose erection is the first response to stimulation, whether this is physical (kissing or manipulating) or psychic (photographs, erotic films, sexual fantasies, sounds, smells, etc). We go back here to the four phases of sexual response defined by Masters and Johnson – excitement, plateau, orgasmic and resolution.

Erection corresponds to the excitement phase. The penis which, when resting, is small, limp and wrinkled, becomes hard and smooth. It swells and grows – in length from about ten centimetres to fifteen or more, and in circumference from seven or eight centimetres to about twelve.

This phenomenon is due to the rush of blood into the three 'little balloons' inside the penis – the two cavernous bodies and the spongy body. The latter is crossed by the urethra, a duct which assures the passage of the sperm (and also the urine) towards the end of the penis. One part of this duct is in the prostate: this is the prostatic urethra. In a few seconds, the penis rises and points forwards and towards the abdomen. The glans, which is at the tip of the penis and hidden by a fold of skin – the foreskin – swells and emerges as it takes on a deeper colour, a dull reddish or violet pink, depending on the individual. The meatus dilates and opens slightly.

During the second – plateau – phase the penis, which is already completely erect, swells again slightly around the crown of the glans. The man can feel that ejaculation is not far off.

In fact, it will come during the orgasmic phase. The prostatic urethra opens up at one end on to the bladder and at the other end towards the penis. Each of these openings is controlled by a sphincter muscle. Before ejaculation, these two muscles act like bolts and tightly close the prostatic urethra, which now only opens on to the two ducts (called the deferent ducts) that direct the spermatozoons produced by the testicles and on to the seminal vesicles, the glands crowning the prostate that carry the sticky liquid part to the sperm.

The prostatic urethra fills up with fluid produced by the prostate, with spermatozoons carried through the deferent ducts and with the sticky liquid provided by the seminal vesicles. Thus filled with three or four cubic centimetres of fluid and therefore under considerable pressure, it opens towards the bottom, reaching the meatus at the tip of the penis. The fluid is ejected in fits and starts, to begin with at intervals of around eight-tenths of a second. After three or four spurts, the intensity decreases and the intervals become longer – up to several seconds.

After the orgasmic phase, which ends in ejaculation, comes the resolution phase. First the penis loses about one-and-a-half times its volume during erection – and that in just a few seconds. Then it returns to its normal size when at rest and the meatus closes up again.

The scrotum and testicles

The scrotum conceals the male glands – the testicles – which produce the spermatozoons and the male sexual hormones. A muscle called the dartos, found in the skin of the scrotum, plays the role of temperature regulator. It maintains a constant temperature of thirty-five degrees inside the scrotum. This is necessary for the testicles to function correctly. When it is cold, the dartos makes the scrotum retract – and expand when it is warm.

Let us look at what the scrotum does during the four phases we have already discussed – excitement, plateau, orgasmic and resolution.

Under the effect of sexual stimulation the scrotum, which is just multiple folds of skin when resting, swells up with a rush of blood while at the same time stretching and losing its folds. This is the excitement phase.

During the plateau and orgasmic phases, the sexual reactions described above can be accentuated, although this is not always the case.

After ejaculation, during the resolution phase, the congestion of the scrotum disappears rapidly and it adopts its original folded appearance. Depending on the individual, the length of this resolution phase can vary from five up to twenty-five minutes.

The testicles also undergo physiological reactions in the course of the four phases of the sex cycle.

Starting with the excitement phase, the testicles rise in the scrotum. In fact, this is just a partial elevation, which continues as the man reaches the plateau phase. Then the testicles come into contact with the perineum (the lower part of the pelvis which stretches from the anus to the genitals).

On this question, it is interesting to note the observations of Masters and Johnson: if there is no – or only partial – elevation of the testicles, then ejaculation is less profuse.

Otherwise, the testicles increase in size – around fifty per cent – under the effect of the congestion caused by a rush of blood in the stimulated sexual organs.

During the orgasmic phase, the testicles continue in the same state as during the plateau phase. There are, however, some changes in the following phase, that of resolution. The testicles go back to their original size and drop down in the scrotum. The time this takes again depends on the individual and can be anything from five to twenty-five minutes.

The breasts

About fifty per cent of men find their breasts sensitive to stimulation. Towards the end of the excitement phase, the nipples become erect and the areoles swell and turn a deeper colour. These reactions generally last until the end of the resolution phase.

Finally, we should point out that breathing frequently accelerates towards the end of the plateau phase and throughout the whole of the orgasmic phase, increasing from ten to fourteen breaths per minute to as many as forty. Also the pulse rate goes up from an average of seventy-two beats per minute to anything from a hundred-and-ten to a hundred-and-eighty. Pressure in the arteries also rises slightly. Equally, a large number of men transpire profusely after ejaculation.

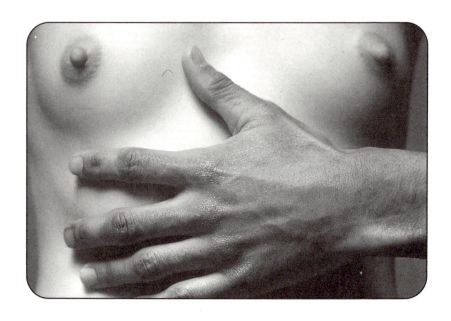

HOW TO SAY IT

At various moments during one's sex life – before, during and after making love – expressing the pleasure, for the man as well as for the woman, reinforces the couple's sensual complicity and strengthens the emotional ties.

At the beginning of a sexual relationship, it is necessary to overcome the embarrassment that people (and especially women) have of speaking about 'those things' – a taboo subject in the majority of families where the rule of silence about sex reigns.

Yet when love is born between two people, they know how to say "I love you" and to express their intimate feelings.

But when the two bodies come together and the couple start to make love, it seems it is more difficult to say openly what they are feeling. Too often timidness and inhibitions prevent the amorous communication that adds even more value to the pleasure both given and received.

"It's barely a year since we got married," writes twenty-one-year-old Amanda, "but what a year it's been. When we made love for the first time, I had absolutely no fear and plenty of desire. I just felt the need for John's body all over. First he caressed me, long and gently, and then he lay on top of me to make love. He whispered such tender words. He told me how soft my skin was, how he adored my breasts and how much my smell excited him. I listened in a kind of trance and the pleasure went right through my body. Afterwards, I fell asleep.

"When I woke up, John was leaning over me, regarding my face. Then he asked: 'Did you like that?' I was struck dumb. It was impossible to let out even a syllable to express what I had felt. All I did was nod my head and I could see that John was upset by my silence.

"It was he who, day after day, each time we made love, solicited the words on my lips and drew me little by little out of my silence and encouraged me eventually to confide in him my innermost feelings.

"Now, I have absolutely no fear at all of talking. I tell John that his penis is beautiful and soft, that he fills me with pleasure, that I love to feel him deep inside me, that my vagina is all damp with the thought of receiving him and that I want him to suck my breasts. When I think that only a few months ago, through false modesty, I kept stubbornly silent . . ."

In the heat of love-making, some slang or obscene words or phrases are often uttered without meaning to be derogatory or degrading. In such moments of intense passion, the man might say "I have a hard-on" instead of "I have an erection" or use the word 'cock' rather than penis or even refer to his partner's vagina as 'pussy'.

The woman may equally use such vocabulary, which is only vulgar when it is used 'cold' and in a context other than that of sexual intercourse. And such words play another role in addition to that of creating excitement. They allow each partner to direct the other, to give indications that will help increase the pleasure at the moment of climax: "Quicker . . . not so hard . . . yes, like that, carry on . . ."

With such words leading up to the moment of orgasm and the groans and cries that respond to a physical need, the final climax – for the man as well as for the woman – is expressed and one should never try to restrain such instinctive reactions.

SEXUAL INTERCOURSE
A LITTLE, A LOT, PASSIONATELY . . . NOT AT ALL

The physical act of making love is one of the 'raison d'être' of a couple. The need of the other responds to an instinct that sublimates love. But here again, sexual personalities differ. Some people are, by nature, generous. Others have lukewarm temperaments.

The question is often posed, by both men and women, about the frequency of love-making. The answer is that there is no norm, save the patterns associated with certain circumstances, such as one's age or state of health.

Some occasions are, of course, more favourable – holidays, absence of children, professional satisfaction – and equally less favourable – stress, unemployment, depression.

Age, for example, does play an important part. From about eighteen and up to one's forties, the sexual urge is at its strongest.

According to a recent European survey, the success rate for intercourse is 76 per cent among those aged between thirty and forty-nine.

From the same survey, of the hundred people aged over twenty who were interviewed, forty-seven said they made love at least once a week, sixteen once a month, seven up to four times a year and thirteen less than once a year.

The French magazine *Marie-Claire* has published the following figures: 8 per cent had intercourse less than once a month, 23 per cent two or three times a month, 24 per cent once a week, 31 per cent two or three times a week, 12 per cent four or five times a week, 1 per cent once a day ... and 2 per cent never.

These statistics simply prove the fact that people make love a little, a lot, passionately or ... not at all, thus confirming the wide differences in habit between individuals.

"I am thirty-two," writes Cyril, "and have been married for seven years. Fiona and I now have sex on average once a week. For the first two years we found we just couldn't satisfy each other; as soon as we were together in the evening, we made love. Then the children arrived and we found we had less time and were necessarily more preoccupied. In brief, our sexual activities were restricted, as a result of which we both suffered from frustration."

This is, of course, a classic case which often confronts couples. It started with youth, passion... making love as often as possible. Then, although neither lost their appetite, a pattern of life became established which was admittedly satisfying but also restricting. As a result, often their sexual relationship no longer took first place.

The risk here is that, as time passes, sex can become less and less important. People start to put it off on the basis that there is always tomorrow and that there are plenty of years ahead. Thus the ever fragile thread of love becomes frayed.

Daphne, who is thirty, expressed her concerns:

"Is it normal to have sex only once a month or even every five or six weeks? It has been like that ever since we knew each other. Yet William is the most tender, the best of companions. As soon as he gets into bed, however, he does the crossword, he reads and then he sleeps. He seems very happy like this, but I remain always hungry for love."

It is not abnormal to have sex just once a month. In fact, as we have seen, this is the case with between 8 per cent and 16 per cent of couples. But this may well not satisfy a young girl with a sensual temperament, as appears to be the case with Daphne. William, on the other hand, seems to be perfectly happy. And herein lies the problem. Partners do not have the same libido. This is true when it comes to appetite . . . or sleep . . . or, indeed, sexuality. There are always those who need more than others.

What should one do when there is a difference in the sexual drive between two people? We believe it is up to the individual concerned who, like Daphne, remains hungry to ask for and encourage sex, to stimulate the partner with caresses and to express clearly the desire for love.

It is rare for any normal individual to resist such obvious advances and not to regain the taste for such pleasures. The woman must not confine herself to a passive role. She has as much right to sexual pleasure as the man and can – and must – seize the initiative. She must be bold in her approach – to want and to be wanted. Her happiness and, indeed, that of the man she loves depends on it.

A quite different case is that of Elisabeth and Gavin. He talks about their situation thus:

"We have been married twenty-five years now and for twenty of those we were making love almost every day, during which time the pattern did not change. Believe me, we were madly in love with each other, always in good health and were lucky enough to want for nothing. The only black spot in our lives was that Elisabeth was never able to have a child.

"We are now in our forties and still in fine form. But there has been a change. Elisabeth has started to reject my advances under a range of pretexts: migraine, her sick mother and so on. It has been more than a month, now, since we last had sex together, despite all the tenderness I have shown her and all my efforts to draw her closer to me. Is this situation normal?"

For twenty years this couple has had plenty of good fortune. It is quite exceptional for love to manifest itself for such a long time through daily sexual intercourse.

So what is happening now?

Elisabeth has gone through the pre-menopause phase, which has brought about some hormonal changes involving a reduction in libido and the erotic function. Such problems can be very quickly and successfully sorted out with treatment prescribed through a gynaecologist.

We should add as a final point here that the barometer of desire is the only guide in the matter of frequency of sexual intercourse and that there is no established rule in this area, which is controlled by natural instinct and chance.

PREGNANCY AND LOVE

In the case of normal pregnancy, a young woman's desire to make love does not go away and, in fact, she can still realise it. Her sexuality can continue to blossom. However, plenty of couples worry about this and abstain from the sexual act because they are afraid that the erect penis is going to 'hit' the back of the vagina, against the foetus, thus risking some damage.

Such fears are quite unjustified. The vagina has, in fact, a perfect 'bolt-hole' – the cervix, which protects the uterus itself, the cavity in which the foetus develops.

In the centre of the cervix is a miniscule hole, which measures only two or three millimetres in diameter. Throughout the period of pregnancy the neck remains completely closed. It only opens at the moment of delivery, when the hole expands to a diameter of ten or eleven centimetres, allowing the baby to pass through it.

The pregnant woman is obviously well cared for by her gynaecologist, who periodically checks that the cervix is behaving correctly. It is only if the doctor decides that the cervix has lost its firmness and has become slightly open that he or she will recommend that there should be no further sexual intercourse. But normally this only happens in about 10 per cent of cases.

Sarah recalls her experiences:

"When I became pregnant for the first time, my husband John started to treat me as something precious and fragile. He told me not to exert myself and to be sensible and rest quietly. He kissed my hands, my feet, my hair... but, despite the fact that he was usually so fiery and amorous, he never went any further as if he was frightened

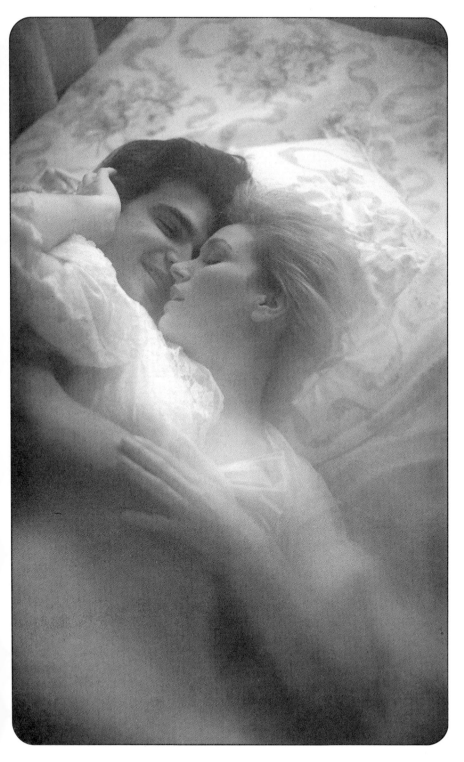

of 'breaking' me if he tried to make love. For my part, I was really desperate for it!

"Finally I spoke to John about it and he admitted to me that he was, in fact, afraid that by making love he might harm the baby and perhaps even deform it in some way. To reassure him completely, I asked him to come with me to the gynaecologist. He was able to explain to my husband that not only was there absolutely no risk to the baby, but also that sexual intercourse was a privileged moment in the life of a couple and that the feelings it produced were completely beneficial."

From the start of pregnancy up to the third month, it is possible to use all the various positions. But when the stomach becomes prominent, one must give up all frontal positions and those that involve the partner putting his full weight on top of the woman, as these are uncomfortable for her. This means using those positions where the man places himself behind the woman and where they are lying together side by side.

It is possible that the discomfort of the first months can affect the pregnant woman's interest in having sex, because she is totally taken up by what is going on inside her.

Such was the case with Pauline:

"At the start of my pregnancy, I suffered so much from nausea and vomiting that I felt completely out of sorts and I really had no wish to indulge in all those things that I enjoyed before – that is to say, the caresses, love-play and having sex. My husband did not complain, accepting what he called my 'whims'. I thought the fact of carrying a child had totally changed me and that, in future, I would be a mother rather than a wife! Happily, towards the end of the second month, the sickness disappeared and I rediscovered the desire for my husband."

There is another subject that preoccupies pregnant women. Some are worried about the strong uterine contractions they experience during sexual intercourse and particularly at the moment of orgasm.

If this happens, one should consult the gynaecologist. An examination will determine whether these contractions result from a change in the cervix. If this is the case, the doctor will advise on the question of making love, usually recommending that this is done more gently and slowly.

THE PREGNANT WOMAN'S REACTIONS TO SEXUAL STIMULATION

The important research carried out by Masters and Johnson on the female's sexuality during pregnancy offers an interesting analysis of the reactions of the breasts and the internal and external genital apparatus to sexual stimulation.

During the first three months of pregnancy, the breasts increase in volume, swollen by a venous congestion. The veins then start to show on the surface of the skin and the areoles become tumescent. Under the effect of stimulation – through caresses both manual and oral – the size of the chest grows even more, provoking an extreme tension which the woman can find quite painful. The nipples and the areoles are more particularly sensitive.

During the following six months, the breasts continue to develop up to a third more than their usual size. But sexual excitement does not make them swell any more. Nevertheless, the nipples become hard and the areoles tumescent. During this period, the pregnant woman does not generally find any caressing of the breasts more painful.

The reactions of the internal and external genital apparatus to sexual stimulation correspond to the vaso-congestion of the pelvis, provoked by the presence of the foetus. Excitement again increases this vaso-congestion.

It has been noted among a large number of pregnant women that the sexual appetite increases towards the end of the first, or the start of the second, three-month period – an urge that continues almost to the end of the pregnancy.

We know that the first indication of desire in the woman is the lubrication of the vagina. This happens between ten and thirty seconds after an effective stimulation. With pregnant women, this lubrication is sometimes affected by the massive hormonal production caused by the pregnancy and can thus be more or less plentiful.

Under the effect of excitement, there are other changes in the genital apparatus of the pregnant woman. The outer lips are congested with blood, as are the inner lips which increase to two or three times their normal size. The vaginal passage is equally congested with blood, but its walls remain supple and, as with a non-pregnant woman, it lengthens and stretches to receive the penis.

At the moment of orgasm, where the subjective sensations occur around the pelvis and involve more particularly the vagina, the clitoris and the uterus, the pregnant woman feels the contractions as usual, that is to say every eight seconds or so, with a minimum of three and a maximum of fifteen repeats.

However, during the last three months of pregnancy, the normal uterine contractions already described can become spasmodic – but in the majority of cases without any damage to the foetus.

After sexual intercourse and orgasm, it takes a certain time – around ten to fifteen minutes – for the vaso-congestion in the genital organs to subside. With those women who have already had several children, this can be as much as forty-five minutes. Obviously this does not impede the women's pleasure at the moment of orgasm.

It is important to note that while this overall picture, drawn up from the observations of Masters and Johnson, has some informative value, it does not necessarily apply to every pregnant woman. Reactions can vary according to the effects of individual psychological or physiological factors.

SEX AFTER CHILDBIRTH

Sexual intercourse can be continued once the woman has finished discharging blood – normally two or three weeks after childbirth. However, this period is not really sufficiently long enough for restoring full sexual relationships.

The woman who has just given birth is often very tired – due to the attention she must give to the baby and the sleepless nights interrupted by regular feeding.

If, at the moment of childbirth, it is necessary to make a cut in the vulva to enable the baby's head to pass through (an operation known as an episiotomy), sexual intercourse is for a while afterwards painful and women have then a tendency to avoid it.

Otherwise, with breast-feeding, the ovaries no longer produce the amount of oestrogenic hormones in the vagina necessary to give it its suppleness, tonicity and lubrication. In the majority of cases, four or five weeks after childbirth orgasm is less intense and shorter. But, at the end of eight to twelve weeks, the woman recovers her full sexual capacity.

Among so many others, here is one testimomy from thirty-year-old Josanne:

"I have now had my third child and can confirm that pregnancy does not last nine months but more like a full year, because during the three months after childbirth couples don't return to a normal sex life.

"After each birth, I felt tired, overwhelmed by everything there was to do after having a baby – in short, I suffered real depression. The occasions when I reluctantly agreed to make love were unpleasant and sometimes painful. It was only with time – in my case between three and four months – that the desire and pleasure returned."

It is important, throughout pregnancy and the three months or so after, that each takes into account the psychological reactions of the other. When the woman is afraid of having sex, then there is a risk that the husband can feel rejected. If there are no medical contra-indications to sexual activity, the couple must speak frankly to each other about the problem.

The single fact of facing it openly together can be enough to dispel the fears of a pregnant woman. If these continue, the gynaecologist should intervene to explain that they are unfounded and equally that it is difficult to impose months of abstinence on the male partner.

In the case where there are real contra-indications to sexual intercourse, the couple will have to resort to caressing each other tenderly and lovingly in order to satisfy their natural desires.

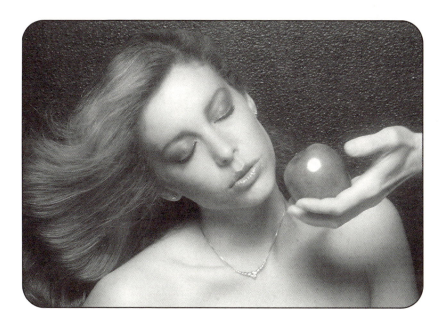

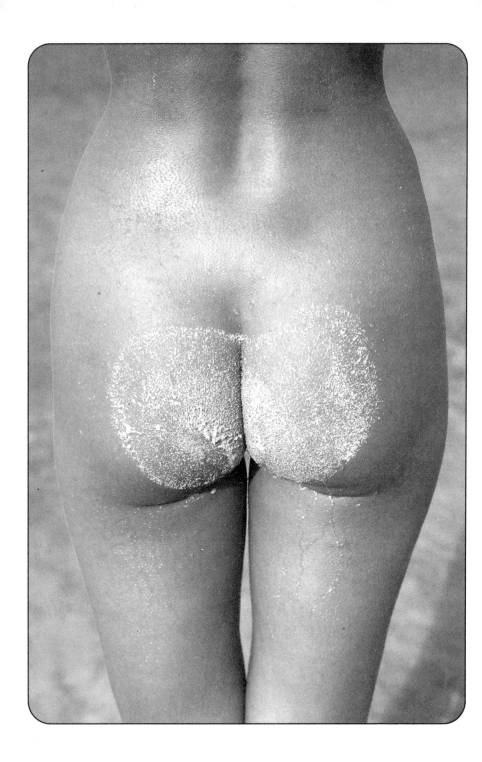

THE SOURCES OF EXCITEMENT

In different forms, through imagination as well as in reality, these feed the sexual appetite

FANTASIES: YOUR SECRET GARDEN

"Imaginary scenario where the subject is present and which represents, in a way more or less distorted by defensive mechanisms, the fulfilment of a desire and, in the last resort, of a subconscious desire."

Such is the definition of fantasy given by Laplanche and Poutelis in their book *The Vocabulary of Psychoanalysis*. In more simple terms, it is an imaginary situation that gives vent to one's desires.

Let us illustrate these definitions with some testimonies.

Steven, who is thirty-five, writes:

"Since adolescence, each time I masturbate or have sex, the same image comes to mind. It's like a real piece of cinema in my head and never fails to excite me.

"I see a young slim girl with long blond hair and completely naked. She has her back to me and I cannot see her face. She is running along the beach with a greyhound beside her. It is a real picture of freshness and purity, up to the moment when a man appears wearing a very tight wetsuit which highlights his swollen penis! He throws himself on the young girl (at which point I am at the height of excitement), pushes her on to the sand and lies on top of her as she struggles – and for me it is orgasm.

"Each time the details are exactly the same. I never tell this to my partners, who find me a marvellous lover and put my amorous exploits down to their own charms."

Twenty-two-year-old Julie recounts:

"It began a year ago. Alex and I have been married for two years. Our love-making has been strong from the start. When we had sex, I thought of nothing else but the pleasure I was experiencing, the sensuous feelings that ran through my whole body.

"Then I became pregnant, which interrupted our love-making during the last five months. For three months after our child was born I was very tired and had absolutely no interest in having sex – or any desire, for that matter. My baby was the only thing that counted. Alex tried to caress me, to excite me, but failed to budge me from my maternal preoccupations. As a result he was suffering; I could see that.

"Finally I talked to my gynaecologist, an amazing young woman. She told me that I had to create a total void in my head when Alex made his approaches and to fill this void with provocative thoughts and fantasies. For example, I should try to imagine that it was my favourite actor who was touching my breasts. Or that I was trying on in front of the mirror all the silk lingerie I dreamed of owning and caressing my body through chiffon, satin or crêpe de Chine. Or even that I was the 'belle of the ball' to which all the dancers in turn made love passionately.

"Such suggestions made me smile. I just didn't think I had the ability to dream up such situations, which appeared to me far more suited to the imagination of a young romantic heroine. Nevertheless, I let such ideas work away in my head and, after a while, I began to have erotic thoughts at the most unlikely moments – while doing the cooking, for example, or when washing my hair. Then, when Alex started making advances and put his hands on me, I felt a slight excitement and didn't push him away.

"Finally, I managed to create my own fantasy after an advertisement on the television which always caught my attention and which I never missed when it was on. It involved a handsome, brown-haired man in a dinner jacket offering an alluring young female a box of chocolates tied up with a large ribbon. The woman was sumptuously dressed in a red satin evening dress, naked at the shoulders and the waist taken in with a wide belt fastened at the small of the back. While she pulled on the ribbon to unwrap the box, he undid the satin belt. In the advertisement, of course, everything stopped there. But in my fantasy, with me being the ravishing beauty, the dress fell in a heap at my feet and my handsome lover knelt in front of me to kiss my vagina.

"Now, each time I try it, my fantasy works. And thanks to it I have rediscovered my taste for pleasure and the desire for my husband."

Everyone has fantasies . . . young girls in full bloom, adolescents in puberty, the most modest of women and the most faithful

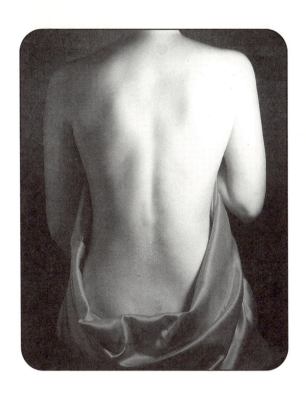

of men. They are made up of snippets of our life, of images, of emotions, of frustrations, of pleasures, of desires. They represent our most intimate secrets, often hidden deep in our subconscious.

It is possible to 'read' a fantasy and to find its roots. In certain cases it is a matter of psychoanalysis, in others simply a matter of psychology.

Let us look at a few examples of fantasies and see what they tell us.

ANDREA AND THE MEN IN CHAINS

Andrea, a twenty-six-year-old secretary, has been married for four years. At work, she had to put up with open advances from her boss, particularly when her husband Thomas was away on business, which happened regularly.

Finally, on one occasion, she gave in to her boss's sexual harassment. Fortunately that seemed to satisfy him and, from then on, he left her alone.

As a young and very sensual woman, Andrea suffered not only emotionally but also sexually from her husband's absence. As a result, she masturbated every night when she was alone in bed, but could only reach orgasm by resorting to a fantasy, always the same, which she describes thus:

"It happens in a large circular room, like an arena. On the ground and against the walls there are ten or so men, all naked and in chains. I am in the middle of the room. I am wearing just a gipsy skirt which reaches down to my ankles and, topless, I dance erotically in front of them. I use every part of my body to excite them. They groan with desire and I watch as they all get an erection. I dance faster and faster as I stroke my breasts. Then I slide a hand under my skirt to masturbate. At that moment, back in the world of reality, I explode with a fabulous orgasm. Curiously, I don't need any of this fantasy in order to come when I am making love with Thomas."

If we analyse Andrea's fantasy, we know that to see men in chains gives her much pleasure. There is, perhaps, here the impression that the desire for revenge against her boss imposes itself on her own desires. Still in her fantasy, Andrea equally takes pleasure in exciting men. Thus she reveals a slight tendency towards exhibitionism, in fact quite common among some women. Finally, when she goes to masturbate, she hides her hand under her skirt as if she was ashamed.

We talked to Andrea about this and she told us that, when she was a child, she had what her parents called 'bad habits' and was often punished for them. Today, at the age of twenty-six, she still suffers a feeling of guilt, albeit subconscious, but which expresses itself through her fantasy.

HUGH AND THE FLUFFY TOYS

Hugh is thirty and his wife Antonia twenty-seven. Hugh is a computer engineer, an only son brought up by a very strict mother and does not have an all-consuming passion for sex. He finds making love once a week amply satisfying. That is not, however, the case with Antonia.

Because he loves his wife, Hugh looks at sex magazines to stimulate himself. He has also bought pornographic videos. Such images have stirred up in his imagination a fantasy that has transformed a temperate husband into a passionate lover. He only has to evoke this fantasy to become incredibly excited.

Antonia does not know the reason for this new-found passion. It is Hugh's secret. And it is also the secret of the couple's happiness. We'll let Hugh explain:

"I am in a room with a huge great bed, very low, on which are scattered lots of fluffy toys of all different sizes. I am laid out among them, completely naked. My eyes are blindfolded. I am listening to very gentle, slow music. I sense the presence of someone else in the room and hear the soft sound of brushing silk. I am aware of a woman getting undressed. She approaches me and I can smell her oriental perfume. I get an extraordinary feeling in my body, as hands wearing soft fur gloves caress me from head to toe, lingering on my hard penis. I feel ashamed to be seen in this state by a complete stranger. Suddenly the woman tears away my blindfold and I look into her face ... It is Antonia!"

Fantasies are often like this: clichés fabricated from images seen or sensed, as was the case with Hugh. They are none the less effective and revealing for that. A childhood regimented by an authoritarian mother left Hugh hungry for compassion. The presence of fluffy toys in his fantasies relates to this childhood loss. The fur gloves provide the softness that he never knew. The caresses make sure that he receives his excitement. And his feeling of fear disappears when he discovers that the woman is, in fact, his own Antonia.

RICHARD AND THE AIR-HOSTESSES

Richard, who is forty and director of a ready-made clothes business, makes frequent and long trips abroad by plane. The hostesses make a great fuss of him and he is happy to chat with these friendly and attractive young women. But he thinks above all about his business and not what passes through his head!

Moreover, he has been happily married to Angela for twelve years and he does not, as he puts it, go 'looking for something else away from the home'. In saying this, he is perfectly sincere. Nevertheless there are two fantasies which he experiences each time he makes love.

"I am climbing the steps of the gangway to board a Boeing 747. I am the captain, dressed in uniform with all my shining brass. On each step there is an air-hostess wearing a skirt so short that I can see the top her stockings and the fastenings of her suspender belt. There are hundreds of steps to this gangway, which climbs up to the sky, and hundreds of seductive women who lick their lips with the end of their tongue as I pass.

"When I finally arrive at the top of the steps, I find myself face to face with a particularly beautiful hostess, with a mouth well made-up and her hair in a tight bun. She waves a magnum of champagne in my face which she opens quickly and shoots the wine all over my penis. It is at this moment that I come.

"My second fantasy also involves a plane and an air-hostess.

In this one I am a passenger. A hostess asks me what I want to drink. She leans over me and I get a good look at her breasts. I slide a hand under her skirt. She is not wearing any panties and her vagina is all damp. She carries on serving. I follow her back towards the galley and push her into the toilets. Once inside, I make love to her standing up."

How many fantasies involve air-hostesses! They haunt the erotic imagination of many a man. Richard is just one of them.

These two fantasies, variations of the same theme, are the simple reactions to the desire to have one of these young women, a desire stemming from the preoccupations of work, the fatigue from a long journey, the concern of avoiding complicating life by getting involved in an affair.

But the desire exists – or has existed. The fantasies are evidence of that.

NADINE AND THE YOUNG BLONDE

Thirty-eight-year-old Nadine only reaches orgasm by evoking a fantasy, which has not changed since she masturbated as an adolescent and has continued through eighteen years of happily married life.

"I am walking through the dormitory of a private boarding school for girls. They are all in bed, with the sheets pulled up to the chin. I go from bed to bed, tearing off the sheets to reveal their adolescent nudity. Some breasts are still small, while others are already showing signs of development. And on each pillow is spread a mop of hair, sometimes brown, sometimes blond.

"A diaphanous figure, with breasts white and round and each pierced by an areole in the form of a pink button, golden hair and a silky pubic triangle, attracts my attention. I lean over the girl to suck her nipples, my hands stroke her stomach and my fingers then slide between the lips of her vagina. It's good. It's soft. I explode with pleasure."

Nadine spent four years in a private school, where Angela became her best friend. They told each other absolutely everything, like one does at fifteen. However Nadine had never confided in Angela the desire she had to caress her, to kiss her lips and to wrap their legs round each other . . . Then the two returned home (they lived in different towns) and never saw each other again.

Nadine then met Timothy. They were very happy together. They loved each other. And they got married. Nadine had fogotten

Angela. But she used to come to mind when Nadine made love with her husband.

This fantasy reflects the frustration Nadine felt from never realising the desire she had for her friend.

It is not, however, the testimony of lesbian tendencies. Nadine never again felt the desire for another woman, since she was perfectly happy and content with her heterosexual life.

Fantasies vary, of course, according to human nature and, in this area, the imagination of some people knows no limits. From extreme violence to the most bizarre situations, anything can emerge from these erotic scenarios.

Take Brian, for example. He sees himself viciously whipping a woman who collapses screaming on the ground from his lashes. It is at that moment that he has an orgasm. This man of forty-two is, in real life, courteous and gentle and very tender with his wife, who says of him: "He wouldn't hurt a fly."

Alexandra imagines that her partner is bound hand and foot, entirely at her mercy, and that she stuffs scarves in his mouth before putting a gag on him. At thirty-three, a mother several times over and an excellent housewife, she has never smacked her children or raised her voice to scold anyone. Doubtless it is by way of compensation for her permanent self-control she has to exercise in order to contain the exasperation she must feel in a domestic environment full of little daily problems that, in her erotic dreaming, she plays a dominating and exacerbated role.

Studies have been made of fantasies. Their ingredients are many and diverse, from rape to sado-masochism, homosexuality to multiple sex, deflowering a virgin to exhibitionism. We should repeat that all this happens only in the mind.

Among the most common, there is the fantasy of the harem. The man is a prince and the women dance and undress for him. He then chooses one or two of them and entices them on to his couch, which is covered in golden silk.

Another very frequently evoked fantasy is that of the doctor. His female patient stretches out naked on the consultation couch. Wearing a white jacket and tortoiseshell-rimmed glasses, he conducts a full and thorough examination before brutally having his way with his patient.

Another fantasy involves the married woman who is rich and very beautiful. She has numerous lovers whom she invites into her bed and afterwards to feast at her dinner table. Her husband, dressed as a maidservant with an embroidered apron and his bottom naked, has to wait on them.

We will stop the examples there to make the point that, while such fantasies make up part of the love-making ritual and feed the sexual appetite, they do not always remain just in the imagination. To realise them and include them in one's actual sex life does carry grave risks. Such behaviour can be very destructive and may upset a couple's equilibrium. Of course, if a man fantasizes about pretty young women in frilly underwear, then there is no harm in his wife wearing such items to please him. But where the fantasy involves any form of violence, for example, we cannot advise people too strongly against such practice in real life.

FETISHISM: OBJECTS OF DESIRE

Defined as a fixation for objects associated with pleasure, fetishism is a form of behaviour that incites the individual to look for sexual satisfaction through contact with or sight of certain objects normally devoid of any erotic significance.

Fetishes have always existed. Among primitive people it was believed that such objects possessed magical powers. These included the talisman and the totem, normally not thought to have any sexual connotation.

In 1886 one Doctor Krafft-Ebing, whose work *Sexual Psychopathy* is still referred to today, classed fetishes in five categories, as follows:

1. A part of the body – breasts, hair, hands, feet.
2. A physical particularity – squint, club-foot, pregnancy.
3. An object or material – underwear, shoes, gloves, silk, leather, fur, plastic, rubber.
4. An action – urinating, washing one's private parts.
5. A psychic attitude – submission, domination.

Since this classification was drawn up, morals have changed. But the principles are none the less valuable for all that. Who doesn't know a man who is fascinated by large breasts or terribly excited by touching silk or a woman irresistibly attracted by someone with a commanding character? As for physical deformities, they still have their followers even if today they are generally less appealing. Bandy legged prostitutes don't go without clients!

In fact, we all have to a greater or lesser degree our fetishes which contribute to our erotic rituals, even if these take on a more benign and normal form. They act like aphrodisiacs. Fetishism becomes abnormal when the fetish acts as a substitute for another person in order to achieve orgasm, for example when a man has an erection and orgasm by simply touching women's underwear and has never experienced the real thing.

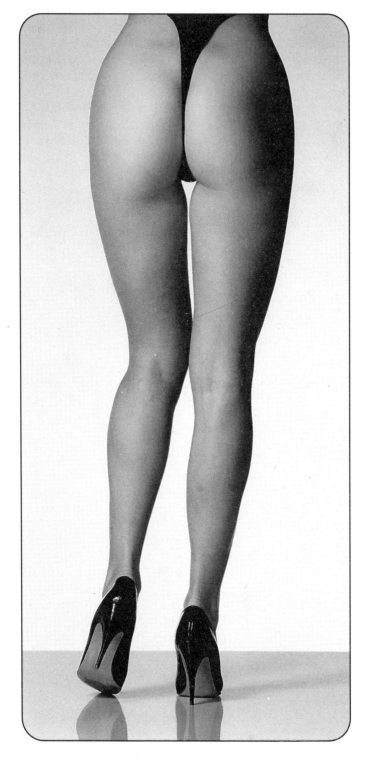

SOME TESTIMONIES

Marianne (age 24)
"Since adolescence, I have worn glasses. I only take them off at night, just before going to sleep. Giles and I have been married for three years. We are both very sensual and make love almost every evening – without glasses, of course. Imagine my suprise when one day, having spent a long time caressing me and at the point of entering me, Giles said firmly: 'Put your glasses back on.' He explained to me later that women who wore glasses always excited him. He even showed me a collection of them he kept hidden in a drawer which he likes stroking."

Richard (age 34)
"The thing I prefer with women is their hair, especially if it is long, black and shiny. I believe I really married Audrey for her hair. Just by touching and breathing in this dark mass and stroking myself with these locks, which are so soft, gives me a stronger orgasm than the one I get when making love. I know this is so, because now I don't have sex any more. It doesn't interest me and I get no pleasure from it. Audrey complains that I only love her for one single part of her pretty little body."

Samantha (age 30)
"My husband is the only one who knows my secret – my passion for those tight black shorts cyclists wear. When I was just a child I followed all the major races on television, full of admiration for these knights on bicycles and fantasizing about their exploits. Then, as I reached the age when I started flirting, boys hardly interested me at all – unless they were wearing those marvellous shorts. One day I went to a sportswear shop and bought a pair, pretending they were for my brother. That evening, in bed, I rubbed myself all over with the shorts. I was twenty-seven when I met Joe and we agreed to get married. We were generally very happy together, but on the sex front we only made love two or three times a month. I decided to take matters into my own hands . . . In fact, physical contact with Joe and his caresses were not exciting me and finally I confided in him my secret passion. He agreed to play my game and now puts on these shorts before joining me in bed. Our life has changed . . . for the greater pleasure of both of us."

VOYEURISM: A CERTAIN LOOK

It is the ban imposed during childhood on seeing or looking at certain acts and situations which breeds just that desire to see, to look, which is essential for the satisfaction of the voyeur.

Forbidden to observe adults in their sexual and sensual relationships, forbidden to touch one's sexual organs because they are 'dirty', forbidden to use certain words... the burden of all these 'don'ts' can influence a child with a particularly sensitive personality and then later, at the age of adolescence or adulthood, a sometimes unhealthy curiosity can creep in.

For true voyeurs, the idea fixed in the head is that of having to see to achieve orgasm. Generally such people are not dangerous because they always keep their distance, isolated in the search for this particular pleasure.

The need to see exists among girls just as much as among boys and can develop in either sex when those involved have been repressed by the restrictions imposed on their natural education.

Just like exhibitionists, voyeurs live a perturbed sexual existence. They feel a deep sense of guilt. Through psychotherapy or analysis, however, they can be helped to rediscover a sexual equilibrium.

Voyeurism also exists in a lesser and very frequent form, which involves the desire to see without necessarily having to achieve orgasm. These types spy, for example, on the neighbours opposite while they are undressing, often using a pair of binoculars to see. This gets them excited and helps them to have even better sexual intercourse with their partner.

There are plenty of people – of both sexes – like this. Their bodies react to the sight of 'hot' love scenes that one sees in practically every film. They cast an eye at the neckline of the woman next to them at a table or direct their attention to the lump that

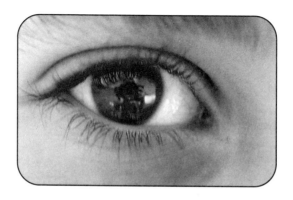

represents the penis in a pair of tight trousers. There is nothing reprehensible in that, nothing abnormal, nothing perverse.

The difference with real voyeurism rests in the fact that such 'onlookers' lead a blossoming sex life, simply fed by such 'stolen' images, while the voyeurs are sexually and psychically immature individuals, incapable of expressing their instincts in a normal context of sensual communication.

SOME TESTIMONIES

Arnold (age 44)
"I had the habit, during my lunch break, to go and eat my sandwiches in the square next to my office. I used to see several young women who went there nearly every day. They tucked into cakes, laughed and whispered in each other's ears. One or two were quite pretty, but it wasn't their faces I looked at. My eyes never left their legs, which they kept crossing and uncrossing, allowing me to get a good look up their skirts. It was extremely revealing. Seeing the scant white panties really turned me on."

Colin (age 38)
"As a book rep, I travel round the country seeing clients and spend many nights away in hotels. I keep in my travel bag a small drill with which I make holes in the doors of the bedrooms next to mine. I get plenty of kicks out of peeping at what goes on inside – undressing, washing, amorous frolics ... I have become an unashamed voyeur. But it's not doing anyone any harm, is it?"

Vicky (age 34)
"I like walking in the woods, not to admire the wonders of nature but in the hope of catching sight of, without being seen, couples in the middle of caressing and making love. I often stumble across this type of spectacle, particularly during the summer."

EXHIBITIONISM: THE BURDEN OF TABOOS

Defined as an obsessional need to display one's nudity and, more precisely, one's genital organs, exhibitionism also exists in less dramatic forms which reveal a simple desire to attract attention or to excite. We will be looking at both these different forms of exhibitionism together.

It is once again to Sigmund Freud that one should look to find the answer to the question: "How does one become exhibitionist?"

The famous doctor who invented psychoanalysis explains that the baby, who has absolutely no notion of good or bad, only looks for pleasure and, in his search to find it, he openly and unguardedly touches his genital organs under the compassionate eyes of his parents who see in this action simply a baby at play.

But this attitude of the parents is going to change. As the child grows up, he will be forbidden from exposing and touching his genital organs. And, to his suprise, he might even be punished when he disobeys. The child is then traumatised and feels such restrictions as an attack on his freedom. By the time he is grown-up, he will find he has an obsessional need to touch and display his genital organs. It is the demonstration of his rebellion against the ban imposed on him and his way of proving that he is free to do what he wants.

Quite clearly, this psychological process does not occur with all children because not all parents, particularly in this day and age, consider it to be a reprehensible act when a baby or young child touches himself.

If one was trying to paint a picture of the typical exhibitionist, the following sketch would probably emerge:

The exhibitionist is generally a timid person who suffers a strong feeling of inferiority and whose sexual life is reduced to masturbating. He has trouble achieving an erection and finds reaching orgasm difficult, too. He remains a bachelor or marries late in life.

Psychologists consider exhibitionism as passive conduct. The exhibitionist exposes his genital organs with the aim of surprising and shocking but attempts no sexual act on his victim, who however regards such a gesture as aggressive and can carry the psychic burden for a long time afterwards.

The exhibitionist frequents the semi-obscurity of gateways, carparks, railway stations, public transport. This is the famous 'dirty man in a raincoat', discreet in appearance, who suddenly plants himself in front of a girl or woman and quickly throws open the front of his coat to reveal his genital organs. Actually it amounts to an indecent assault, which is punishable by law. The exhibitionist is an unhappy person who can only be helped to get rid of his obsession through psychotherapy.

We say that the exhibitionist is an unhappy man, implying that this problem does not exist among women. Of course it does, but such cases of true exhibitionism are rare, no doubt because the instinctive need to show one's sexual organs concerns women less than men and that because of the very nature of the organs. The idea of aggression is linked with the penis and not the vulva.

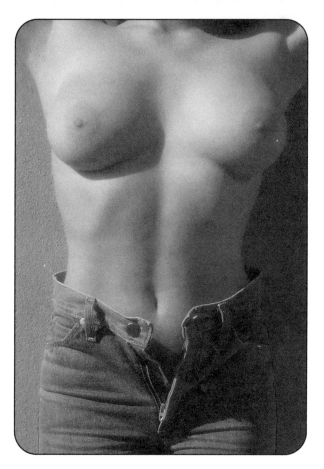

Exhibitionism does not limit itself just to the display of the sexual organs. As Dr Krafft-Ebing states, it also reveals itself in other ways. He listed four basic categories. But that was in the middle of the last century and we will see that today one can add to this.

For Dr Krafft-Ebing, exhibitionism manifests itself "in the exposure of the penis, accompanied by masturbation – or not, as the case may be; in nudity other than that of the virile organ; in the practice of sexual acts in the presence of other people; and in obscene proposals".

All that remains true. But we can extend this to cover contemporary life, which is witness to a milder form of exhibitionism, not obsessional and certainly very common. Cinema, television, newspapers and the advertising industry all make use of nude images, of scantily clad bodies; clothes are designed and created to be provocative; tight jeans emphasize one's sexual organs; shirts and blouses leave the breasts exposed; skirts barely come down below the top of the thighs. One can cite hundreds of examples of everyday exhibitionism, as much among women as men.

"I am twenty-five," writes Margaret. "I am very fashion-conscious and I adore wearing miniskirts and black stockings with lace tops. I wear a tight slip of assorted lace and I take an evil delight, when I get out of a car, in spreading open my legs to show the white of my thighs and let the men guess what there is above."

There you have it! Today's version of exhibitionism. Nothing reprehensible, not even the desire to shock although certainly to please.

Alan also finds pleasure in exhibitionism.
"I am thirty-two and my wife Diana twenty-eight," he tells us. "She is a pretty woman, slightly plump, with angel skin and golden locks. She excites me a lot. I have offered her some adorable naughty underwear that one can easily see through a near-transparent blouse. In black stockings and high heels, she is irresistible. When we go out, we like to pick our spot outside a café in a popular area. Diana crosses her legs so that virtually everything is in view and then the two of us watch as the men pass by. This little game certainly stirs them up. These little displays of exhibitionism really do get us excited."

To conclude, what was considered yesterday as exhibitionist behaviour is no longer regarded as such today. We refer particularly to naked bodies on the beach, bathing costumes that have been reduced to virtually nothing, the practice of nudism, of communal undressing in the changing-rooms of sports clubs ... and so on.

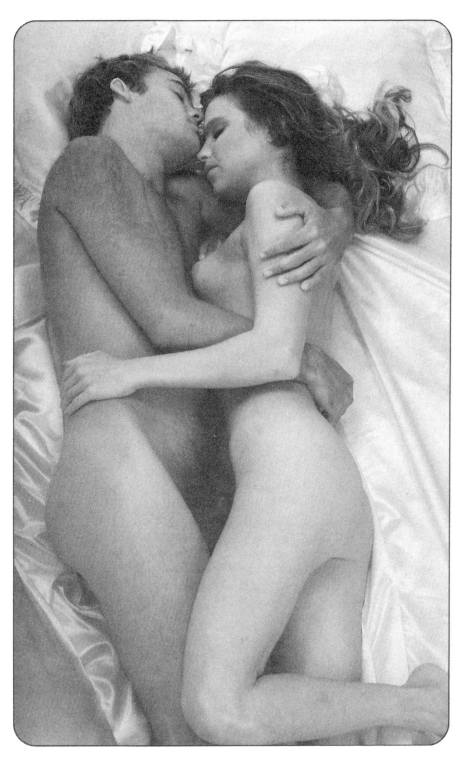

4

LOVE-MAKING POSITIONS

VARIATIONS ON THE POSITIONS OR 52 WAYS OF MAKING LOVE

The sexual potential of each man or woman is infinite and should be developed by practising different positions to provoke different sensations. We all know that monotony leads to boredom and that the variety of positions is a source of excitement which brings with it the discovery of new pleasures.

"Learning to make love is a necessity . . . For a long time, it was said that learning how to make love was an aberration . . . It was to risk chasing spontaneity, the sense of playfulness and the expression of its own fantasy. Fifteen years of clinical experiences have, however, shown us that even nature and instinct need evening classes."

These few words from Dr Gilbert Tordjman, taken from his book *The Profession of Sexology*, underline the fact that the complicity between two bodies and the coming-together of those great desires rely on an apprenticeship in eroticism, which first begins with touch and then the realisation of the sexual act. This must in turn lead to the absolute pleasure – orgasm – and it is essential to regenerate this throughout the life of a couple together.

It is in this perspective that the know-how of love and foreplay plays its part in that wonderful moment of peace and relaxation following the sexual climax.

1 THE MISSIONARY

This is the position most practised in the East – and for a number of reasons. The couple are facing each other so that they can see the signs of pleasure on each other's face. They can also talk to each other, exchange tender words or express their delight by talking about the sensations they are feeling and what their preferences are. Some women particularly appreciate this position, since they do not have to take any initiative and the feeling of being dominated by the man increases their pleasure.

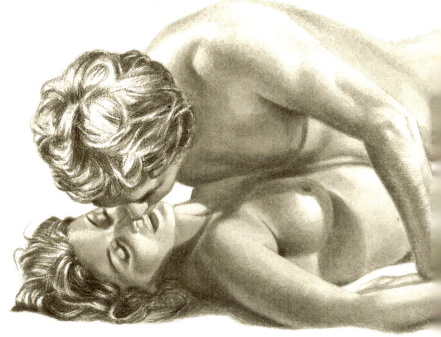

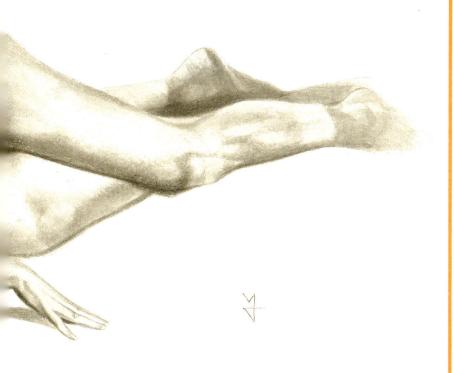

2   THE DOMINATOR

The woman lies on her back with her knees bent upwards, arms along her body and thighs open. The man kneels over her, holds her by the hands and then penetrates her. It is he who controls the in-and-out motion. In this position, the man can at the same time kiss his partner's face and her breasts.

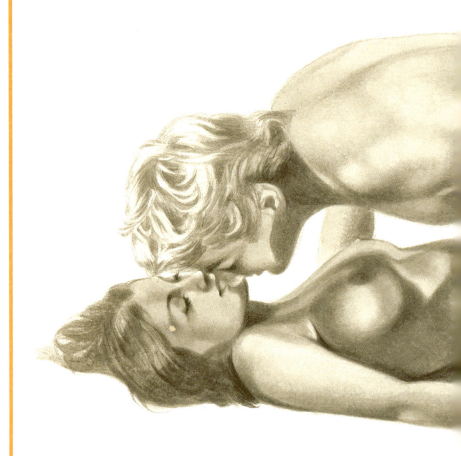

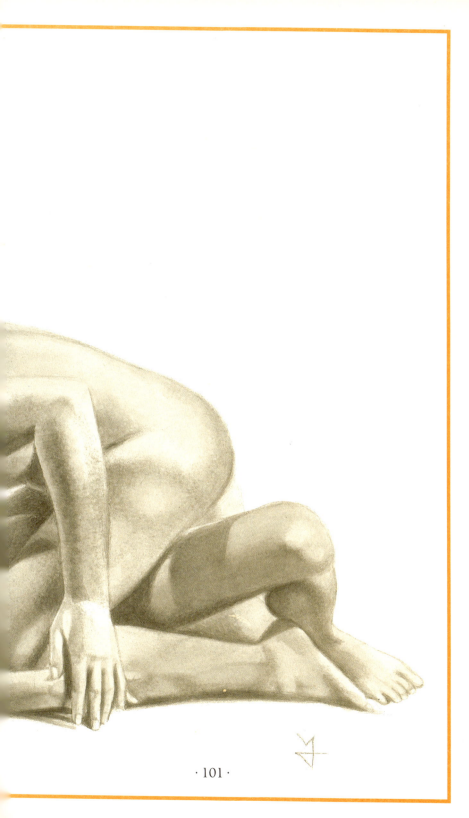

3 THE CAPTIVE

The man lies on his back and lifts up his thighs and bends his knees so that his calves are parallel to the bed. The woman kneels in front of him and puts her hands on his chest, thus impaling herself on his penis. Here the man remains motionless as the woman moves up and down, allowing her partner to see the expression of pleasure on her face.

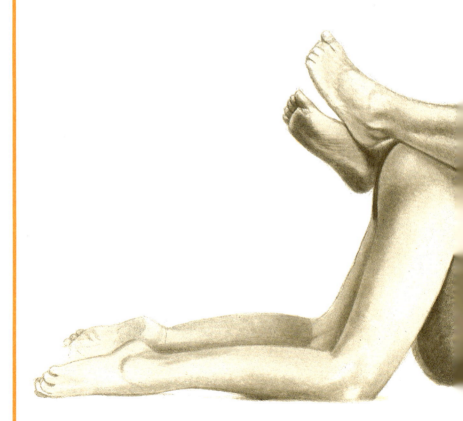

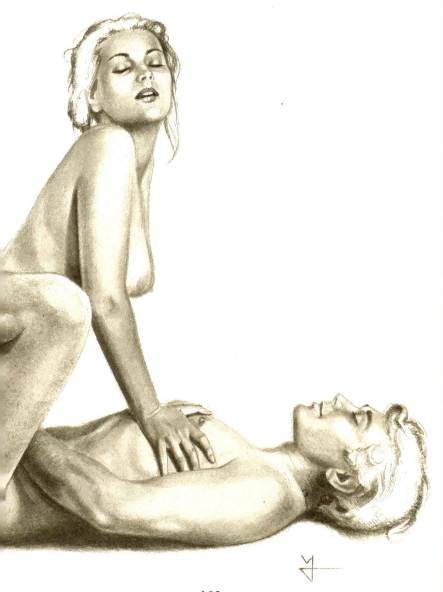

4 THE HUG

The man lies on one side, as does the woman – with her back tucked in to the front of her partner. In this position he can penetrate her while, at the same time, sensually caressing her body – from her breasts to her clitoris.

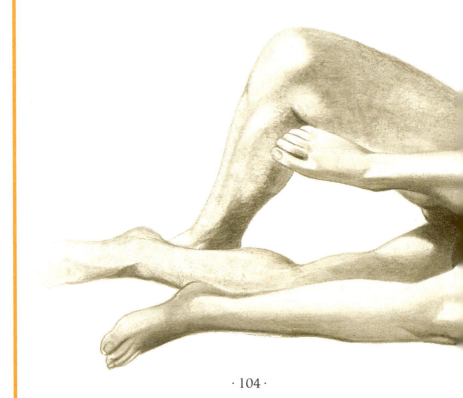

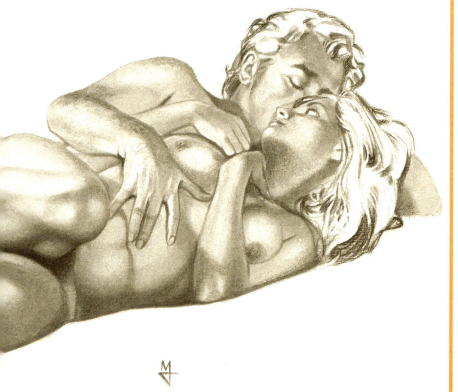

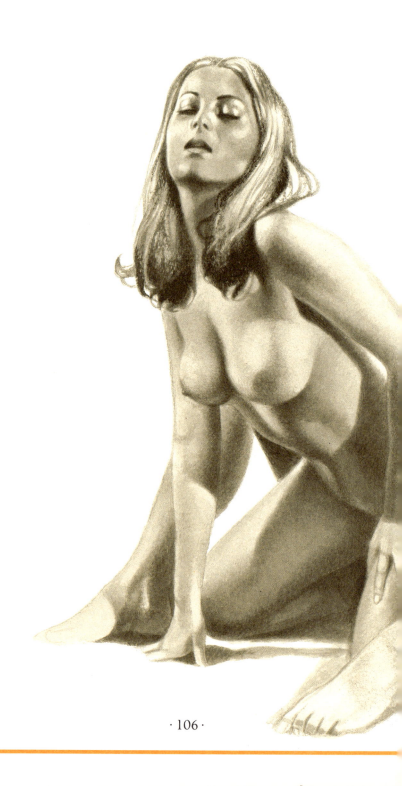

5 THE VOLUPTUOUS

The man sits on the bed and leans back against the pillows. With her back to him, the woman kneels between his legs, leaning forwards and supporting herself with her arms. Her partner can thus enter her, after which she is responsible for the motion. Such a position, where the woman presents her backside, always creates great excitement for the man.

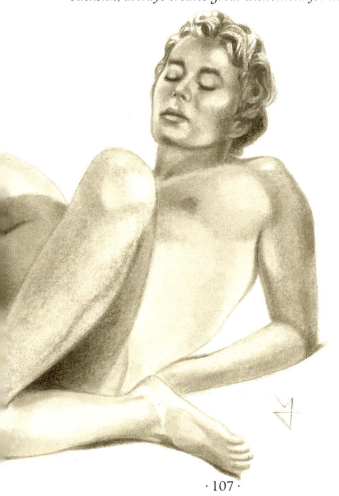

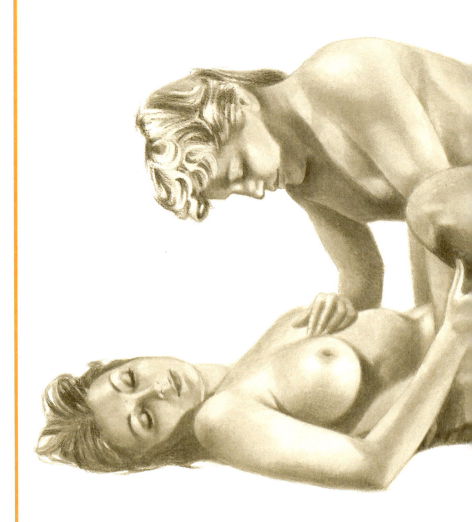

6 THE EXCHANGE

The woman lies on her back, with her knees bent and her thighs open. The man crouches above her as he rides and penetrates her. In this position, the hands are free for mutual caressing.

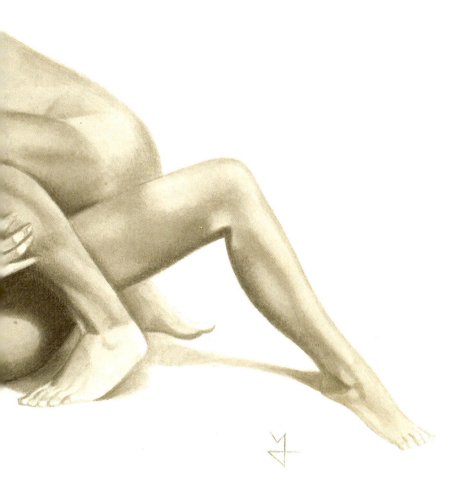

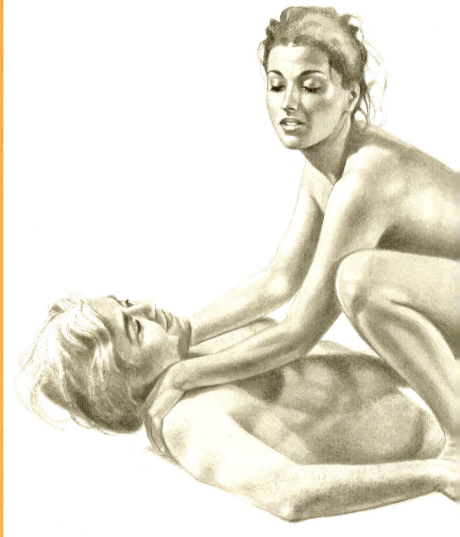

7 THE RIDER

The man lies on his back with his thighs slightly open. The woman then 'rides' him, face to face, with her hands on his shoulders. The man's hands are free to caress his partner's breasts. This is a suitable position for someone with a short penis.

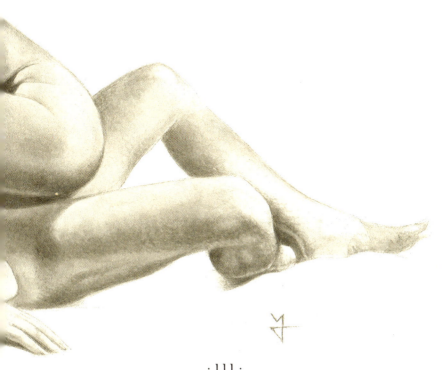

8   THE INTERWEAVING

The woman lies partly on her side, resting on her elbow. The man places himself between her thighs. She bends one knee and puts that leg over her partner's hip, with her heel between his buttocks. He then penetrates her and, during the motion, she caresses his anus and perineum – two very excitable areas – with her foot. Equally, he can tickle her clitoris and breasts.

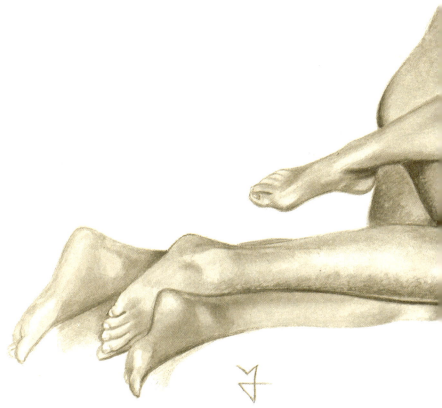

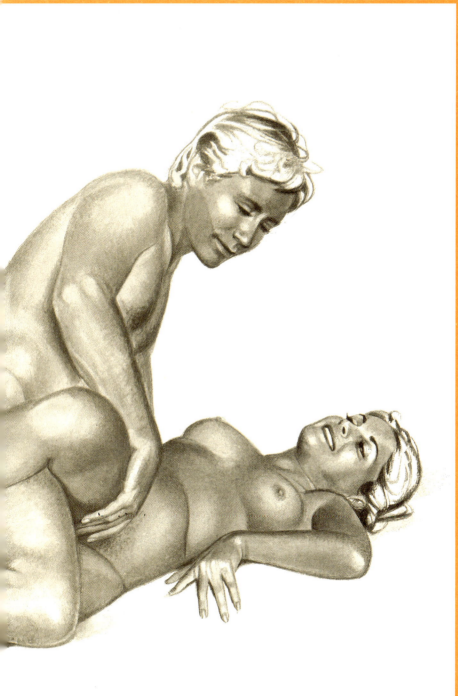

9 THE COAXER

The man sits, leaning on some pillows. His partner sits on top with her back to him. In this position, penetration is very deep. With one hand free, he can then caress her body.

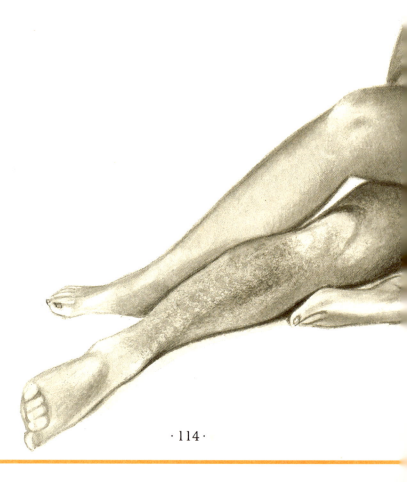

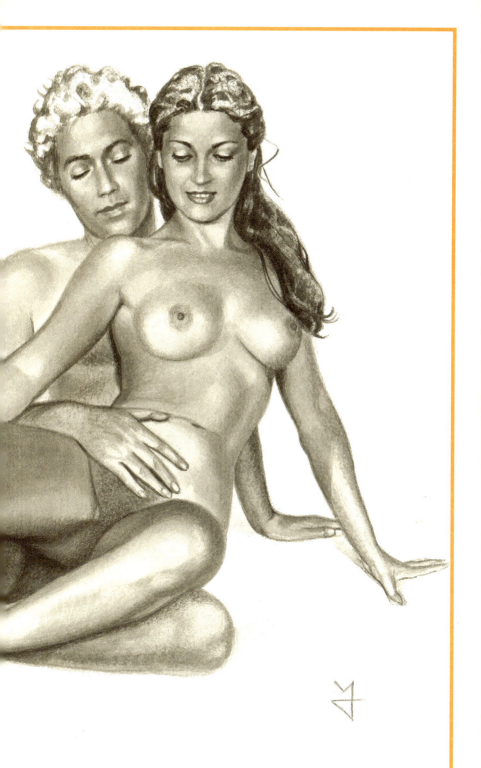

10 THE WRESTLER

The man kneels, with his thighs open. The woman, facing him, sits down on his thighs and allows him to penetrate her. They wrap their arms around each other and exchange deep kisses. In this position, which combines tenderness with sensuality, the woman plays the active role.

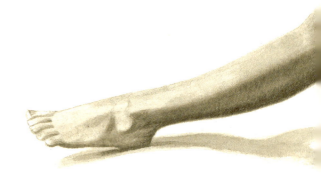

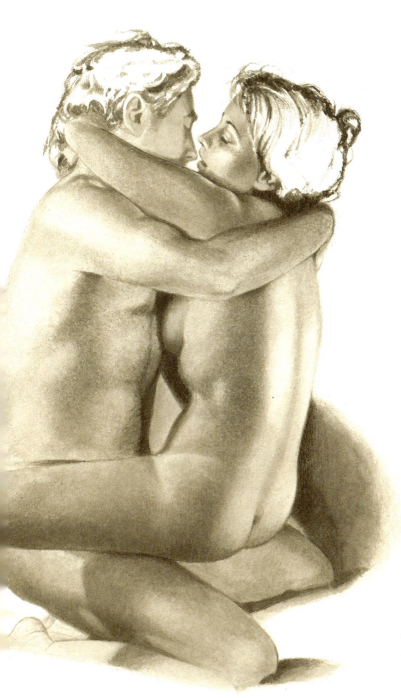

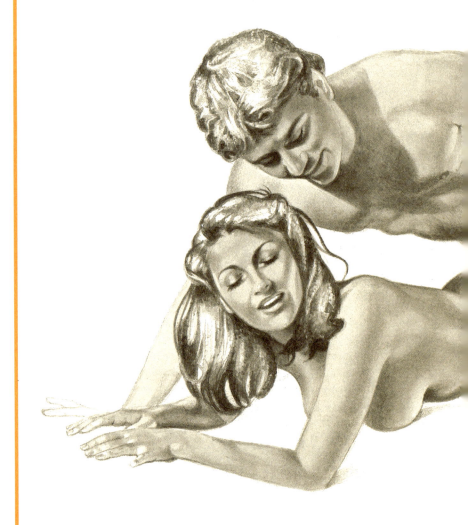

11 THE BULL

The woman stretches out on her front, resting on her elbows, with her back to her partner. He kneels over her, supporting himself with one hand while he 'rides her', using his free hand to manipulate her thigh and achieve the in-and-out motion.

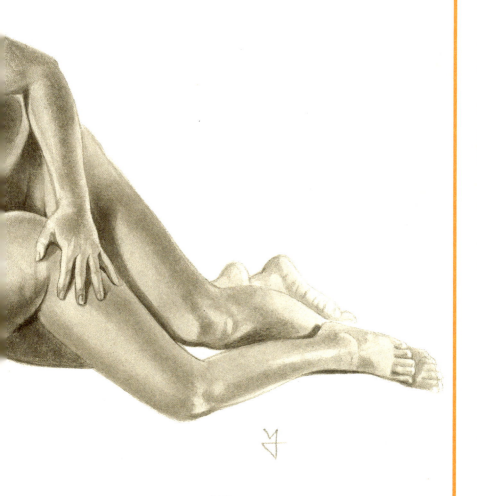

12 THE LOVE TRAP

The man sits with his knees bent and legs open, as he leans against the top of the bed. The woman kneels astride and facing him, with her hands resting on his shoulders. He in turn clasps his hands together under his knees as he works his partner's hips to and fro in the required manner.

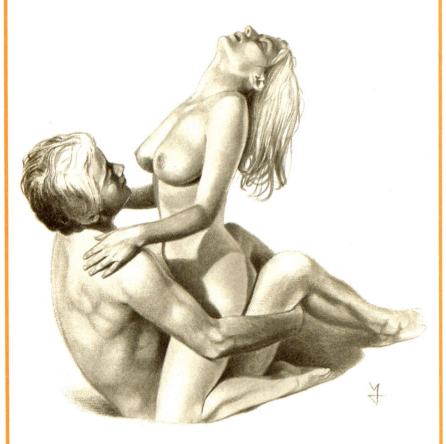

13 THE MASTER

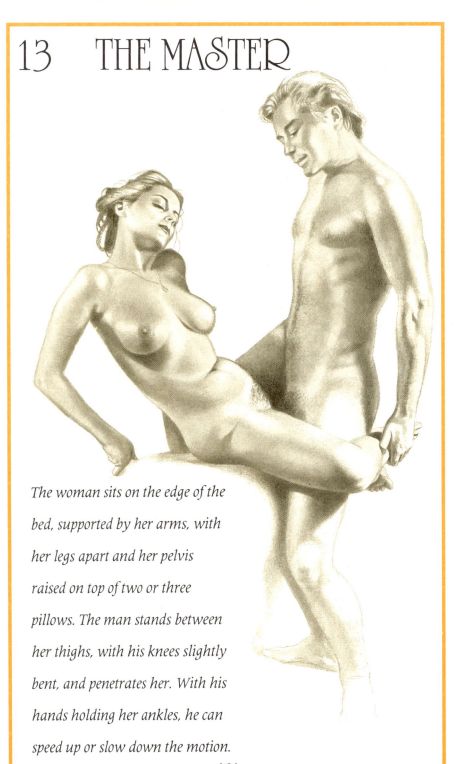

The woman sits on the edge of the bed, supported by her arms, with her legs apart and her pelvis raised on top of two or three pillows. The man stands between her thighs, with his knees slightly bent, and penetrates her. With his hands holding her ankles, he can speed up or slow down the motion.

14 THE YOUNG SHE-GOAT

The woman kneels down on the bed, resting on her arms, and opens her legs. The man sits behind her, with his legs raised and knees bent and supporting himself on his elbows. This position, in which the woman controls the rhythm, allows for deep penetration.

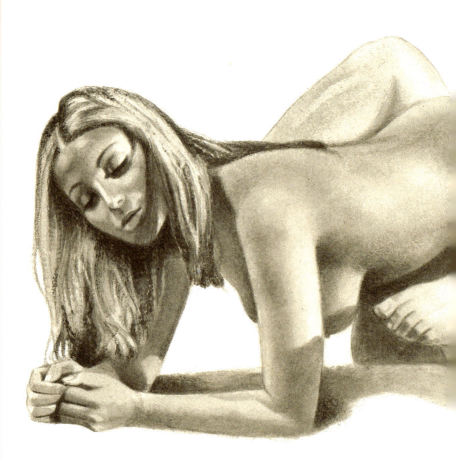

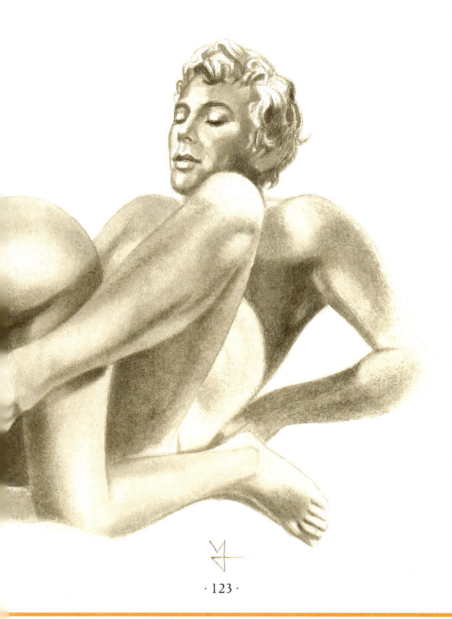

15 THE GATE OF PARADISE

The man kneels down on the bed, resting on his hands. He then leans over the woman, who is lying on her back. She raises her legs and wraps them round her partner's waist. With her hands free, she can caress her breasts and those of her partner.

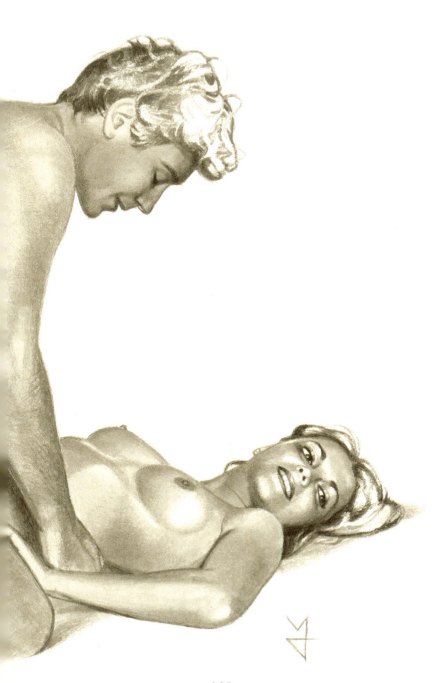

16 THE TROPICAL

The man lies on a narrow surface, with his arms resting alongside his body. The woman sits on top of her partner with her back to him and her legs hanging down on either side. She leans forward, tucking her breasts in between his legs and taking hold of his feet.

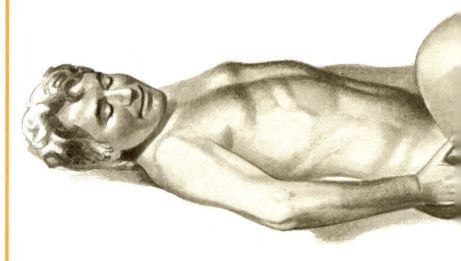

In this position, he can lift her thighs and bottom up and down as he wants, while she caresses the soles of his feet and his toes – erogenous zones for a lot of men. Not only is this position very comfortable for the man, but it also allows him to see his partner's buttocks in action.

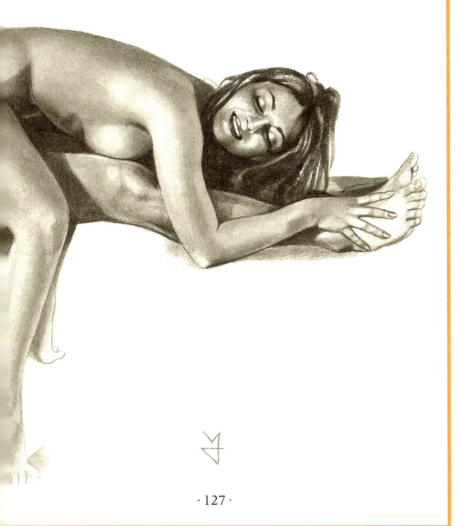

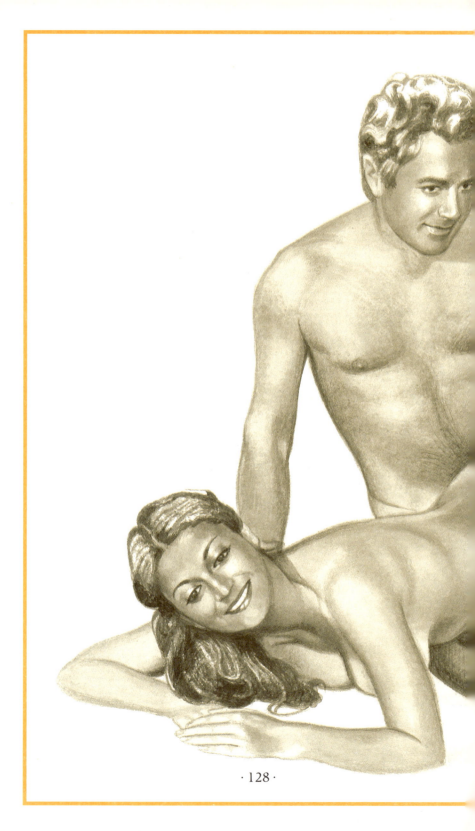

17 THE PIVOT

The man sits on his heels, resting on one arm. The woman lays herself across his knees, with her legs apart. He penetrates her in this position. The two stay still like this. He caresses her with his free hand until the point of extreme excitement. Then the woman starts to move her pelvis up and down in a slow rhythmic action. This position does not allow for very deep penetration and is most suitable for men with a long penis which might otherwise frighten some partners.

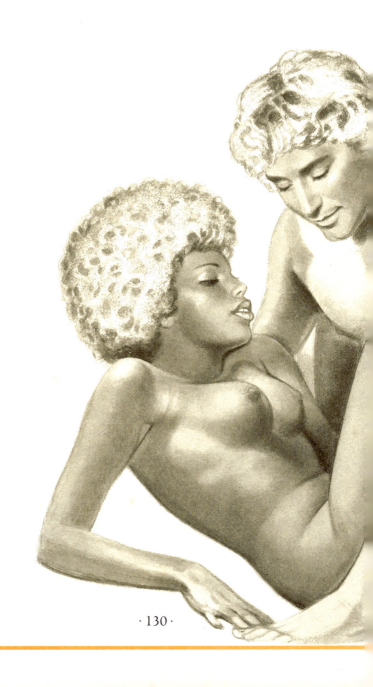

8 THE DOUBLE CAVALCADE

The man sits with his legs wide apart. The woman sits in front of him, supporting herself on her forearms and resting her legs on top of his. He makes the movements as his partner remains motionless. This position enables each to watch the pleasure on the other's face right up to the moment of orgasm.

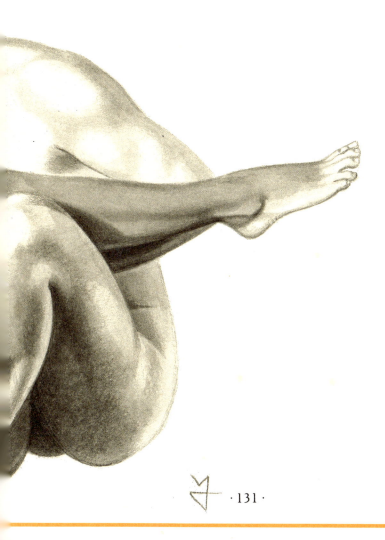

19 THE SUBMISSIVE

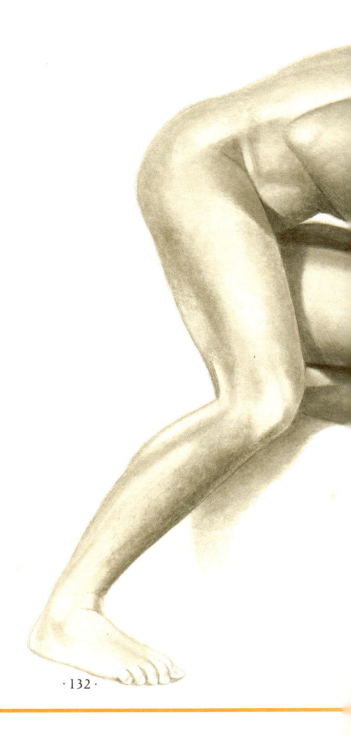

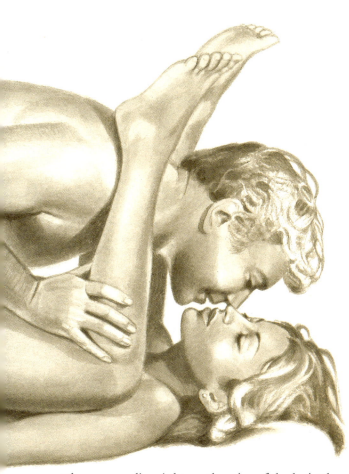

The woman lies right on the edge of the bed. The man stands facing her then leans over on top of her as he pushes her legs back over her body so that her knees touch her shoulders and her ankles rest on his shoulders. As he holds her calves, he bends his knees and enters her. This position, in which the man does all the movement, allows for very deep penetration but does require a degree of agility on the part of the woman.

20 THE SEE-SAW

The man lies back on the edge of the bed, with his legs wide apart, his knees bent and his feet firmly on the floor. The woman gets in between, with one leg over and one leg under his. In this way she can 'ride' him. As they hold each other by the arms, each moves in turn. This position is particularly suitable for those young athletic couples always looking for variety in their sexual activity.

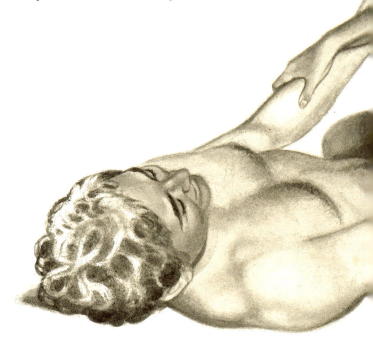

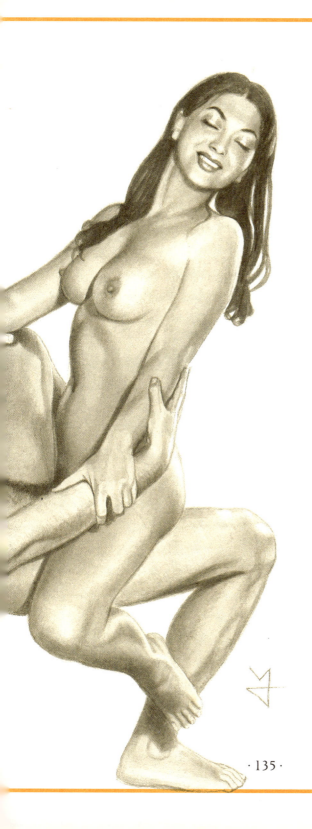

21 THE BUTTERFLY

The man sits on the edge of the bed. Then the woman sits on top of him and, with her legs wide apart, lets him penetrate her. With their free hands, they caress each other.

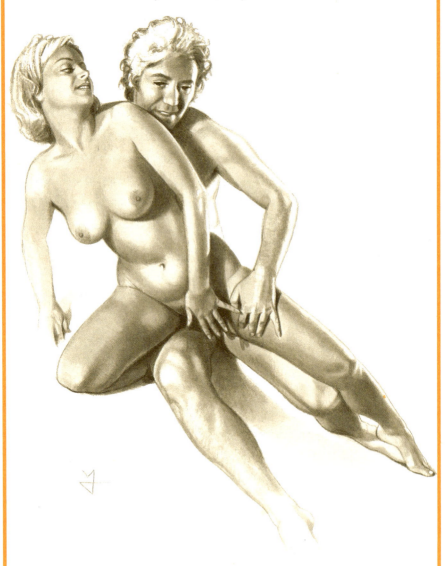

22 THE FACE-TO-FACE

The man and the woman kneel in front of each other. She slides one knee between the thighs of her partner and then lifts her other knee so that her foot supports her on the floor.

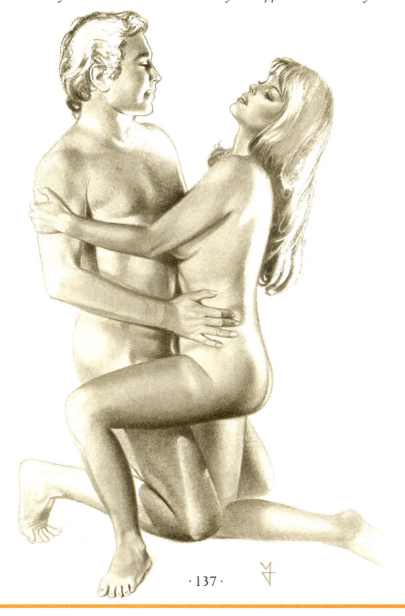

23 THE ACCOMPLICE

Both partners lie on their side, with the man behind the woman. He then lifts up her thigh and places it on his. He penetrates her in this position, which allows him to caress her with his mouth and tongue, particularly around the ear and the nape of the neck.

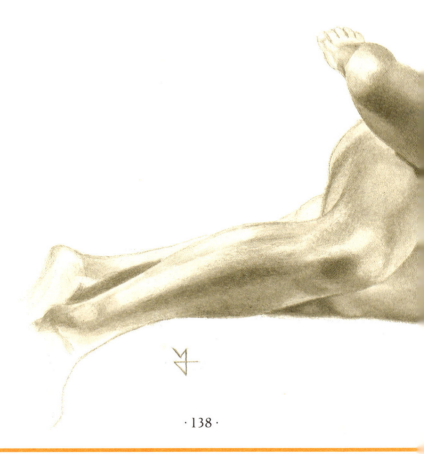

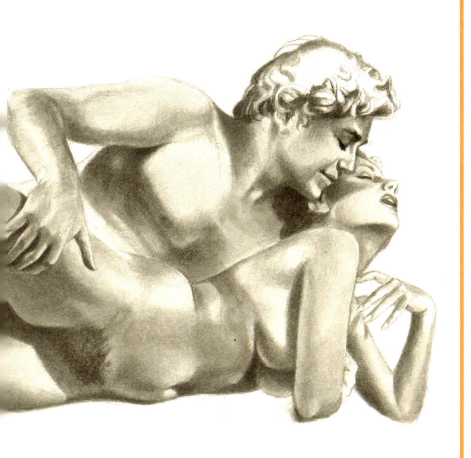

24 THE SOFT SURRENDER

The woman lies on her back with her head resting on her partner's arm and he lies alongside her. She lays her thighs across his. In this position of 'surrender', he penetrates her as he caresses the whole of her body. There are plenty of women who get more pleasure out of such caressing than the sexual act itself.

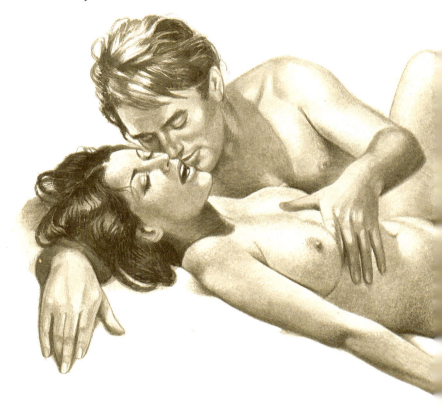

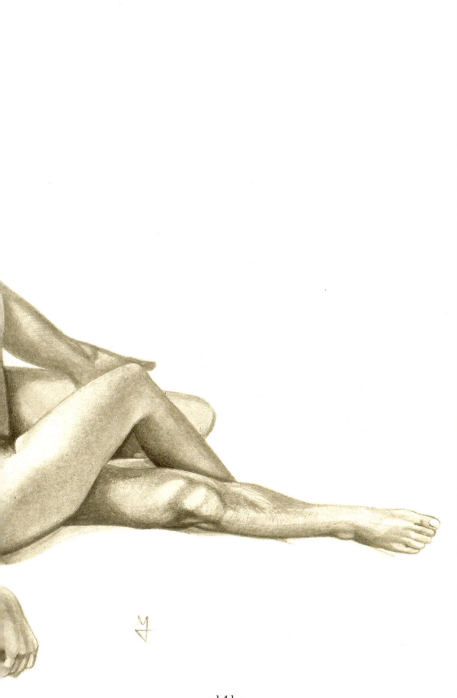

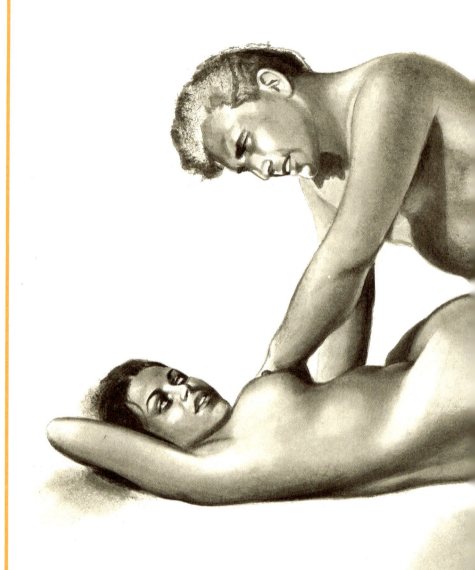

25 THE WHIRLPOOL

The woman lies on her back on the edge of the bed while the man kneels beside her on the floor. By swivelling her hips round, she allows her partner to penetrate her. As he bends over her, he can stroke her breasts.

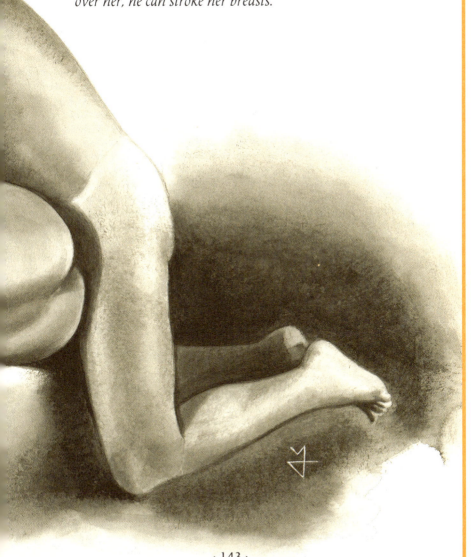

26 THE BOAT

The man sits with his back supported and his legs apart and knees bent. The woman sits between his thighs with her back to him, enabling him to penetrate. Then she crosses her legs over his. She uses her outstretched arms as support while her partner, holding her by the hips, directs the intercourse and, at the same time, experiences a feeling of power.

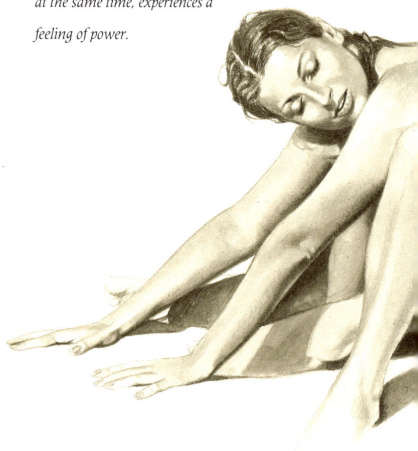

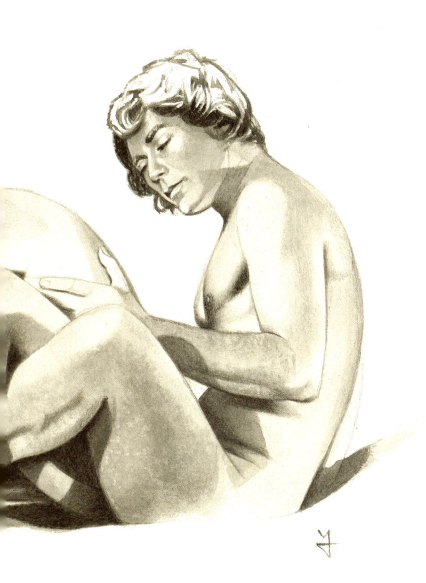

27 THE DOUBLE GAME

Both partners lie on their side, head to foot, with the woman showing her back to the man. The double advantage of this position is that it allows for deep penetration but is not tiring.

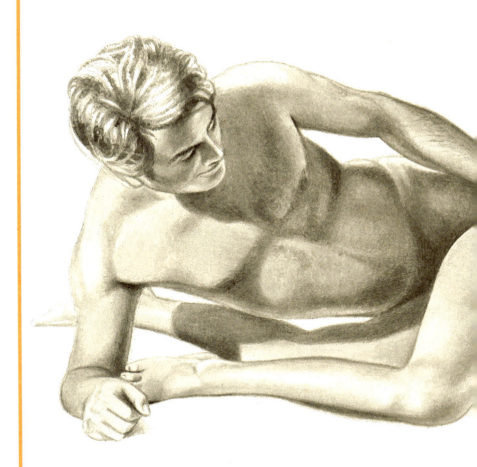

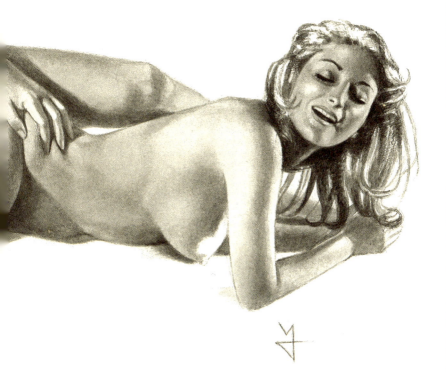

28 THE SHARING

The woman lies on her back, with her arms down the side of her body. The man kneels in front of her and lifts up her legs, which he holds in this position. Then, leaning on the other arm, he enters her and starts the motion, slowly at first and then gradually more quickly.

In such a position, each partner can follow the pleasure expressed on the face of the other.

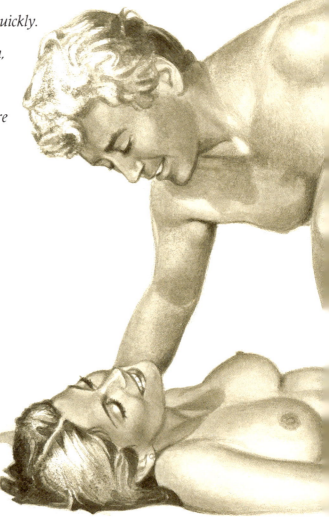

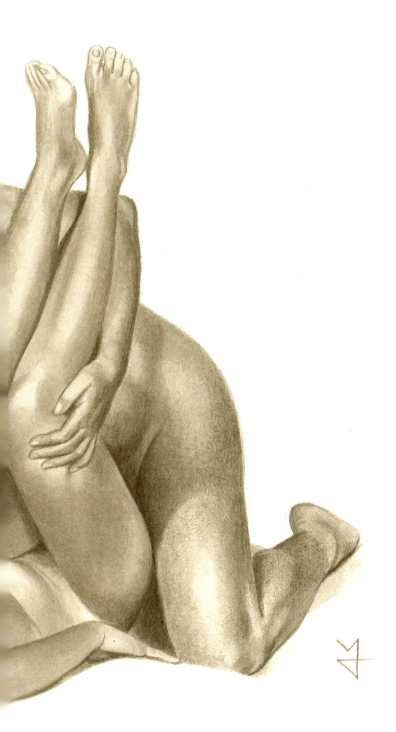

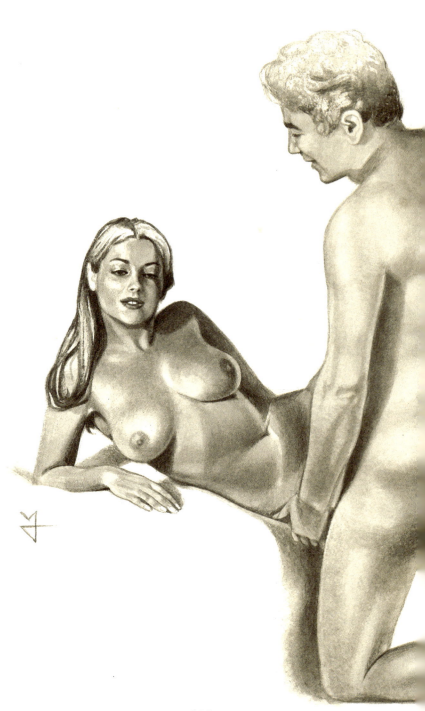

29 THE BIG SHIVER

The woman lies on her side, supporting herself with her elbow and with her pelvis resting on the edge of the bed. She lifts up her thigh to offer herself to her partner, who is kneeling on the floor in front of her. He lifts the raised leg while straddling the other. The contact is thus very restricted – and very exciting.

30 THE AMAZON

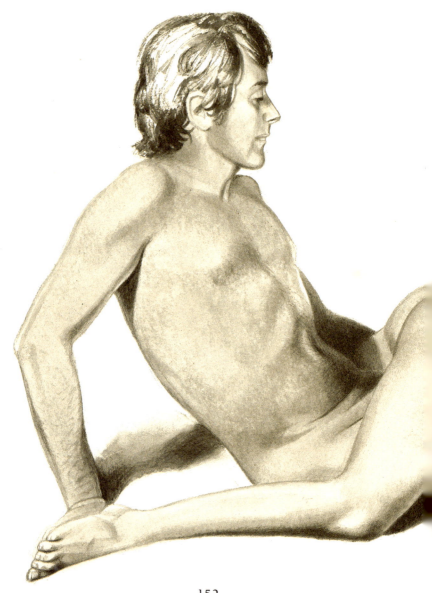

The man sits up, supported by his arms, with his legs stretched out in front of him. The woman, with her back to her partner, 'rides' him, while also using her arms as a support. By bending and then straightening them, she effects the in-and-out motion and, in this position, controls the love-making.

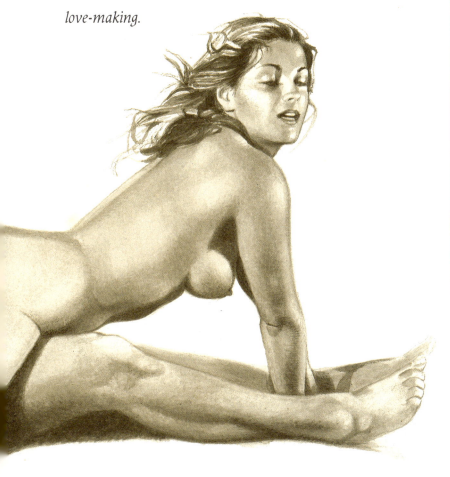

31 THE OPEN FLOWER

The man lies to one side in a half-upright position, resting on an elbow. With her back to him, the woman 'rides' her partner. He in turn can stroke the back of her body while she controls the movement.

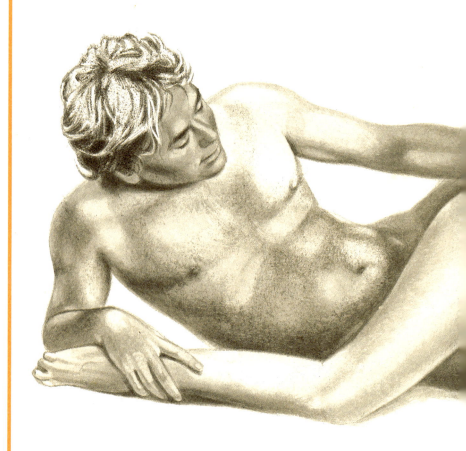

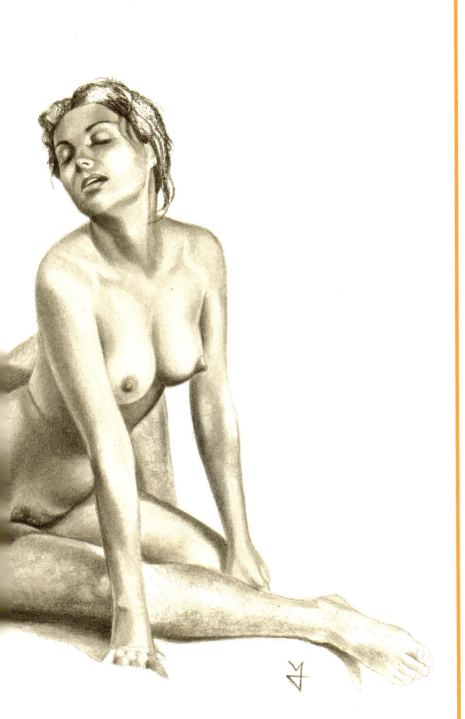

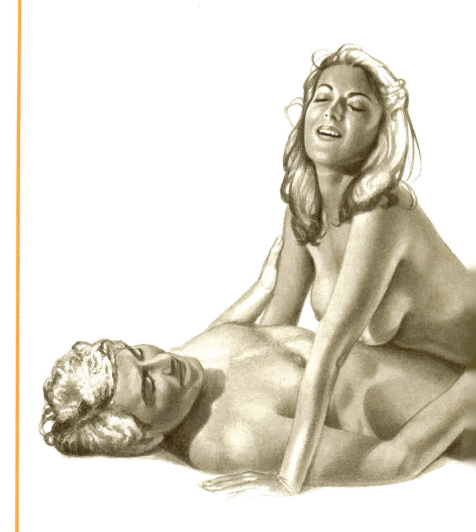

32 THE LONG DISTANCE

The man stretches out flat on his back, with his legs apart. The woman lies on top of him, supporting herself with her arms either side of his shoulders. He controls the motion by holding his partner by the hips and moving them up and down. This position does not require any special effort and enables the couple to prolong the sexual act.

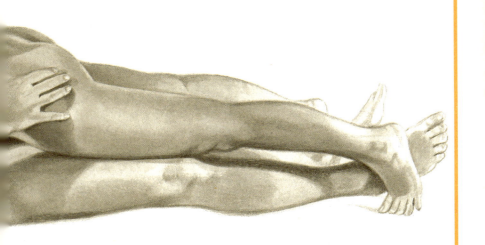

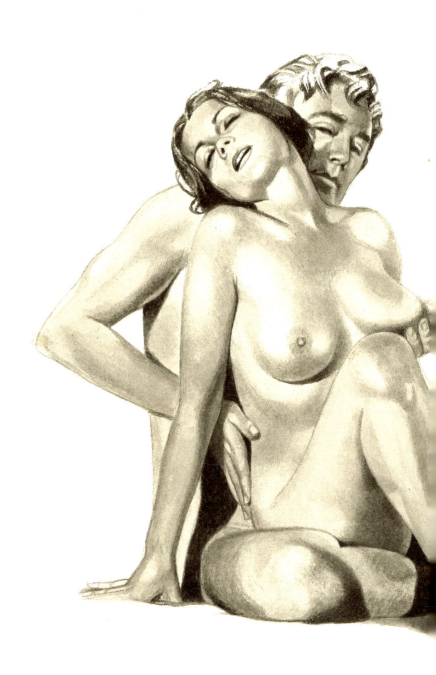

33 THE WAVES OF THE SEA

The man sits upright with his legs apart. The woman impales herself on him as she rests her back against his chest. In this position, the man can caress her breasts and her clitoris, while she makes the necessary motions with her pelvis.

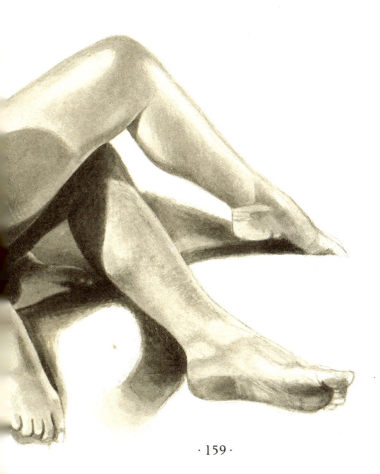

34 THE MISTRESS

The man lies on his back, with his head and shoulders slightly raised by some pillows. The woman sits on top of him and 'rides' him, controlling the rhythm of intercourse through the movement of her pelvis.

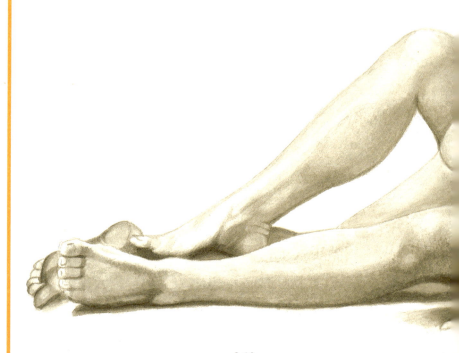

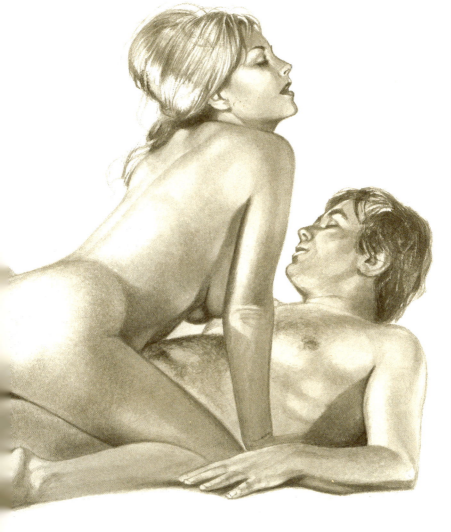

35 THE FIREWORKS

With both partners lying on their side, they fold their legs and tuck themselves together. This position enables the man to caress the woman's bottom, as well as her clitoris and breasts.

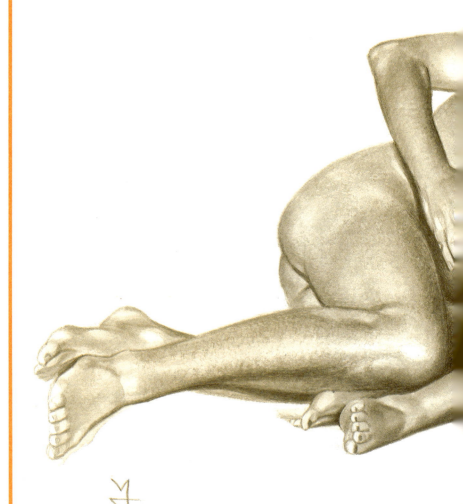

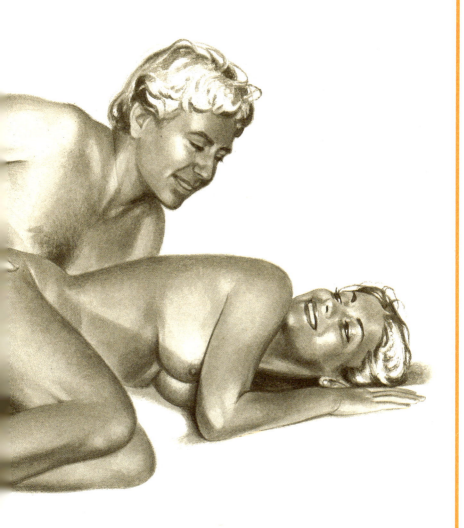

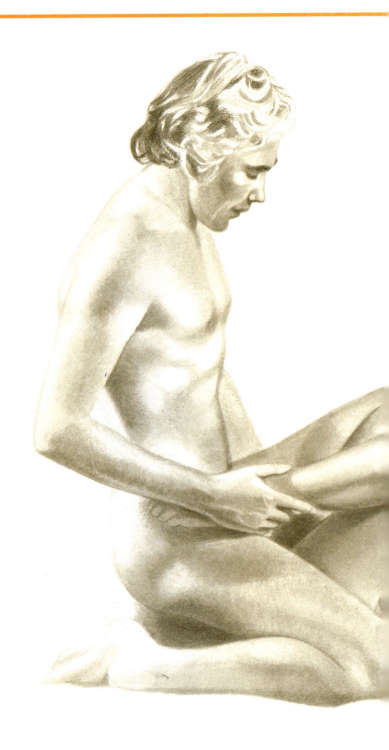

36 THE LOVING HOLD

The man kneels back while the woman lies with her bottom tucked in between his thighs and her knees bent so that her feet rest on his hips. Holding her ankles, he penetrates her, while she caresses her breasts. For deeper penetration, she can lie on a cushion to raise her pelvis.

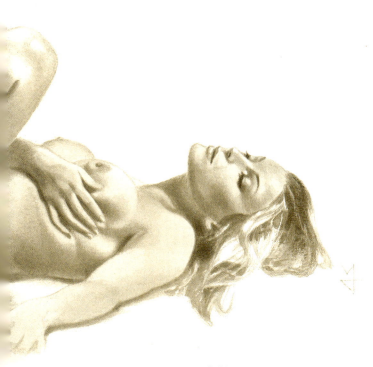

37 THE HOP

The man lies stretched out as the woman, squatting with her back to him, 'rides' him. Supporting herself with her arms, she moves her pelvis up and down under the direction of her partner, who holds her by her buttocks. This position requires the woman to be quite agile.

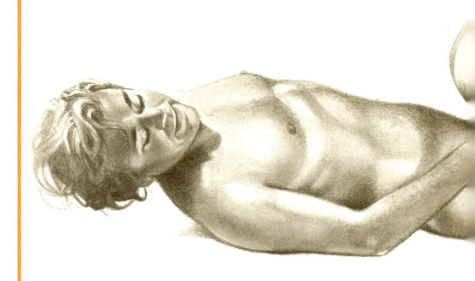

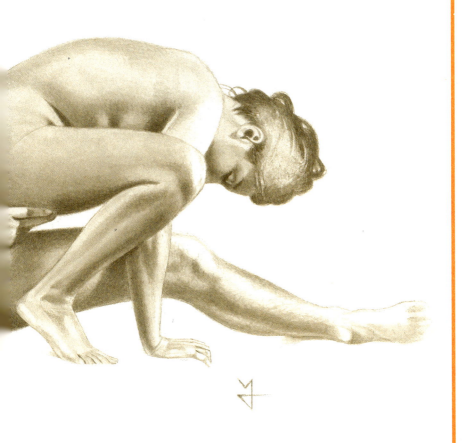

38 THE GEISHA

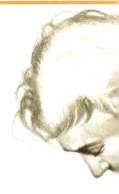

The woman stretches out on her side at the edge of the bed, presenting her vagina from behind to her partner, who kneels beside her on the floor. In this position he can caress the whole of her back, from the neck to the bottom, as well as her breasts, stomach and clitoris.

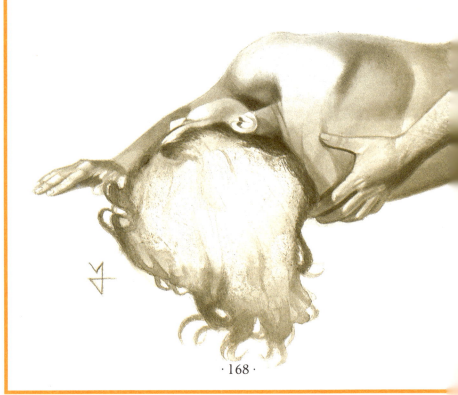

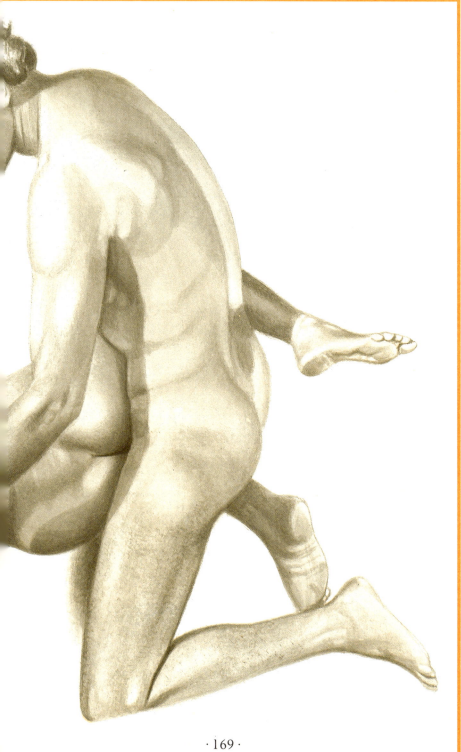

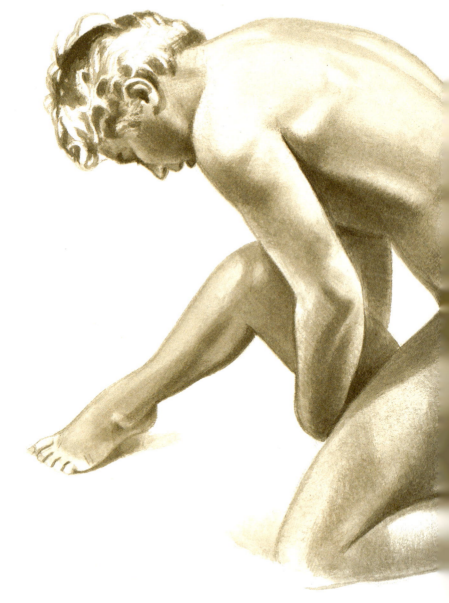

39 THE SENSUAL RIDE

The woman lies on her back and raises one knee. Her partner, kneeling over this leg, 'rides' her. She then raises her other leg, bending it so she can rest it on his back, and holds him by the hips. He in turns holds on to her other leg to steady himself. In this position, it is the woman who controls the motion. By pushing with her folded leg on her partner's bottom and back, she makes him move in and out.

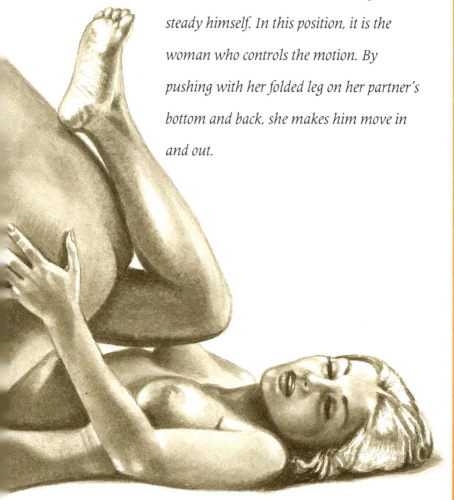

40 THE SPLITS

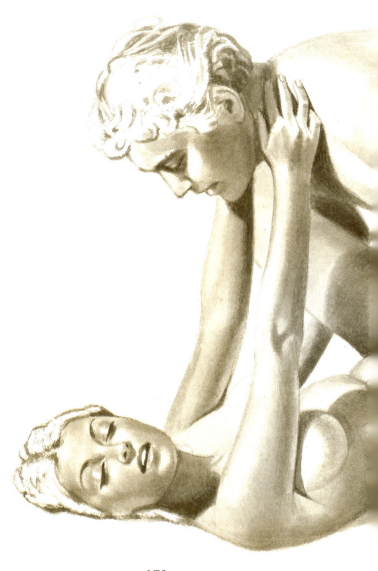

The woman lies on her back, with her pelvis raised by pillows. The man kneels down between her open thighs, which she raises and rests on her partner's arms. She stretches her arms to take hold of his neck and draw him towards her. In this position, penetration is very deep and it is the man who plays the active role.

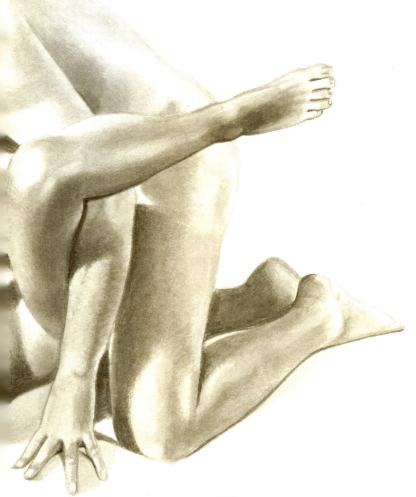

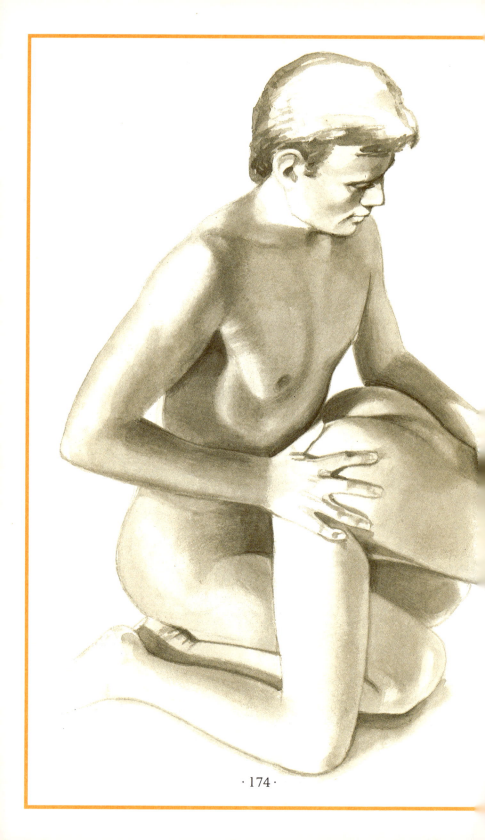

41 THE GREYHOUND

The woman kneels down and stretches forward, resting on her hands, thus offering herself to her partner, who squats down behind her, in between her legs, and penetrates her while caressing her bottom and back.

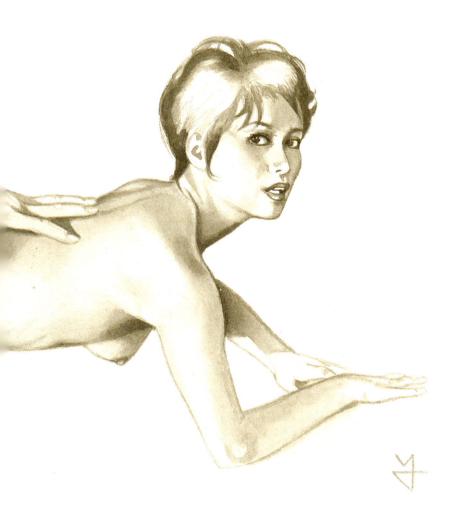

42 THE QUIET LOVE

The man lies flat on his back and the woman stretches out on top of him with her legs apart. She lifts herself up slightly, supported by her arms. In this position, where the man can caress the whole of her back, it is the woman who plays the active role.

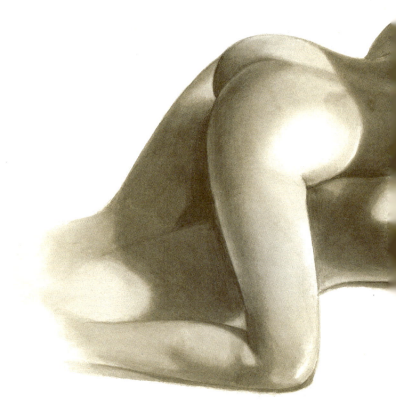

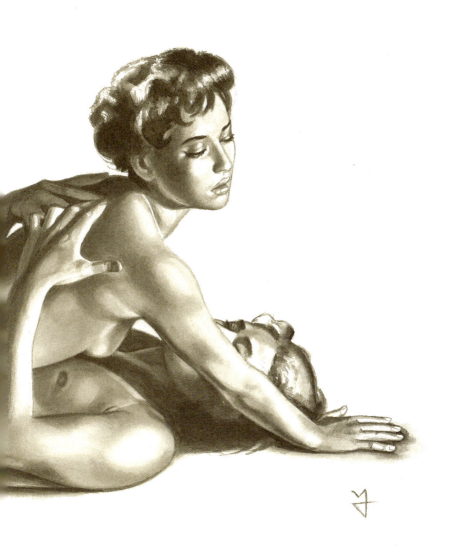

43 THE GAZELLE

With his back slightly raised by pillows and with one leg stretched out and the other raised, the man takes his partner between his thighs. Supported by her arms, the woman bends and stretches to create the in-and-out movement, while the man caresses her buttocks with his raised leg.

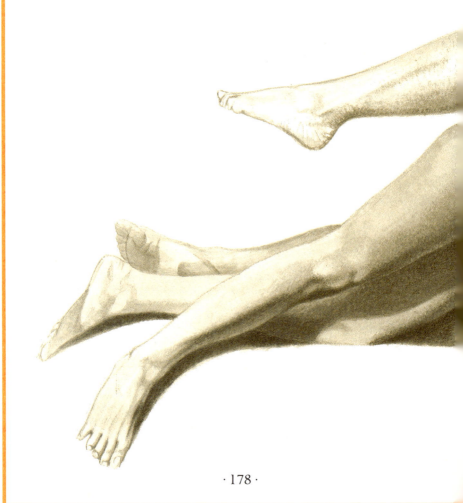

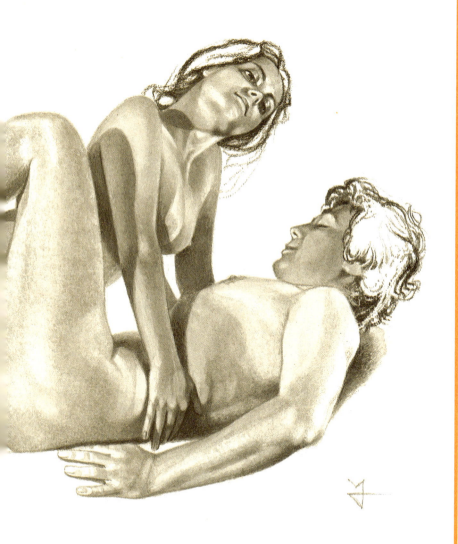

44 THE WATCHING

The man lies on his side, propping himself on one elbow. He then opens his thighs, on which his partner sits down, facing him. He holds her by her heels as she moves her pelvis to and fro in the usual way.

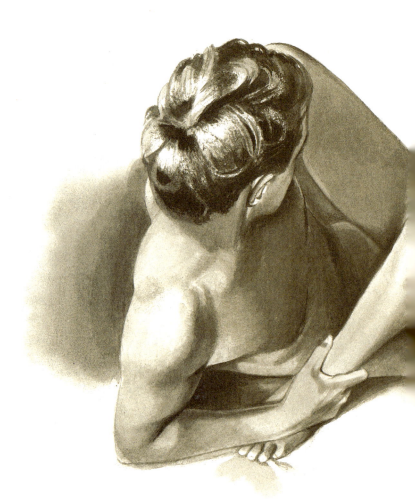

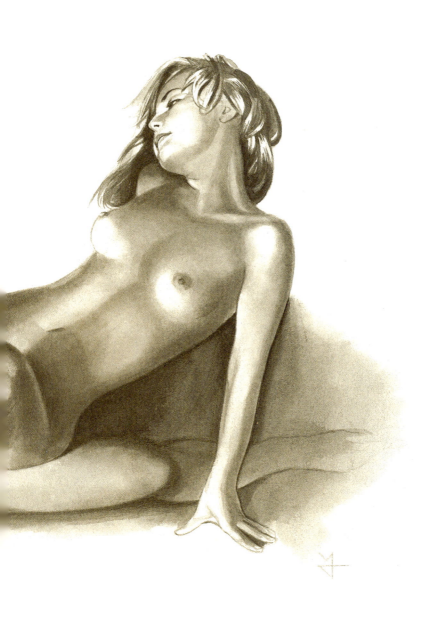

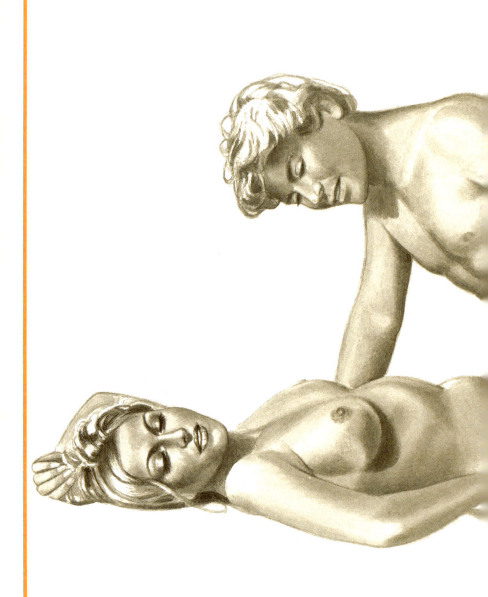

45 THE CARESSING LOVE

The woman lies back on the edge of the bed, her feet resting on the floor and her legs apart. The man kneels down between her thighs and penetrates her, using one hand for support and the other to caress the whole of her body.

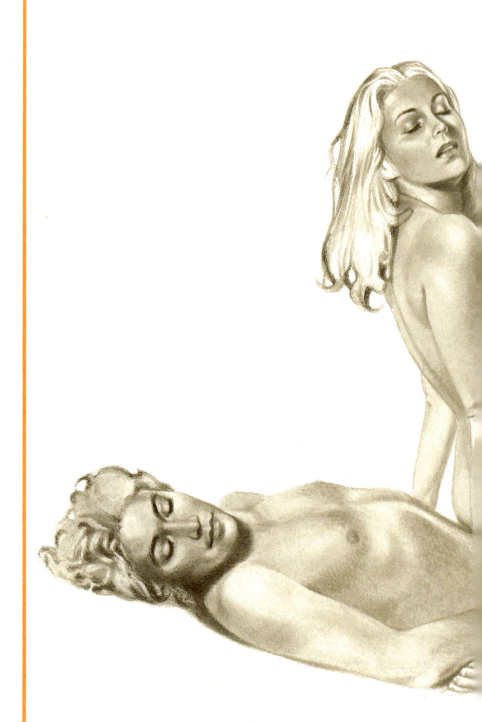

46 THE PRISONER

The man lies flat on his back and the woman, facing away, sits on top and 'rides' him, as she holds him by the wrists. By moving her pelvis up and down, she has perfect control over the sexual act.

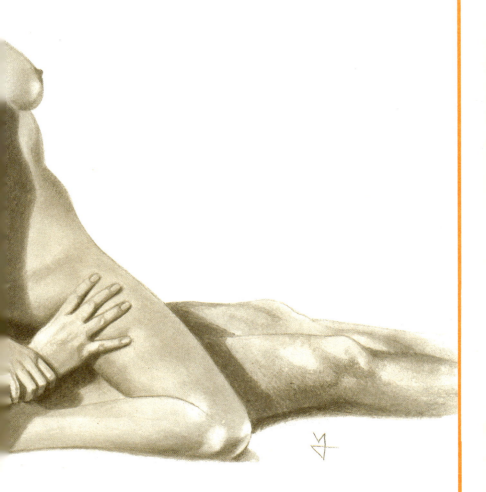

47 THE OFFERING

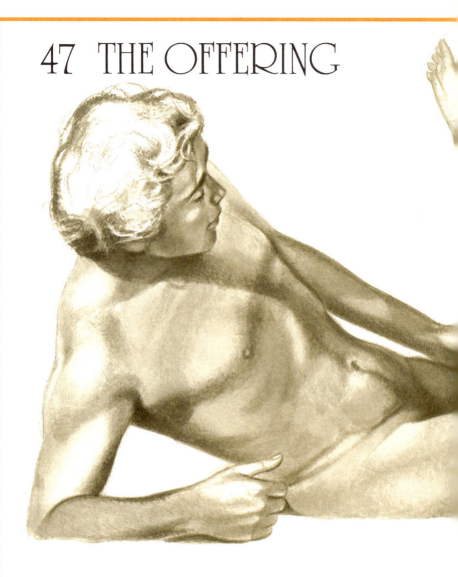

The man sits on the edge of the bed, resting on his elbow and with his legs apart, one foot on the floor. The woman lies between his legs, with her knees bent and raised, as she offers herself to him. This is a position for the start of intercourse. Afterwards the two continue, lying head to foot.

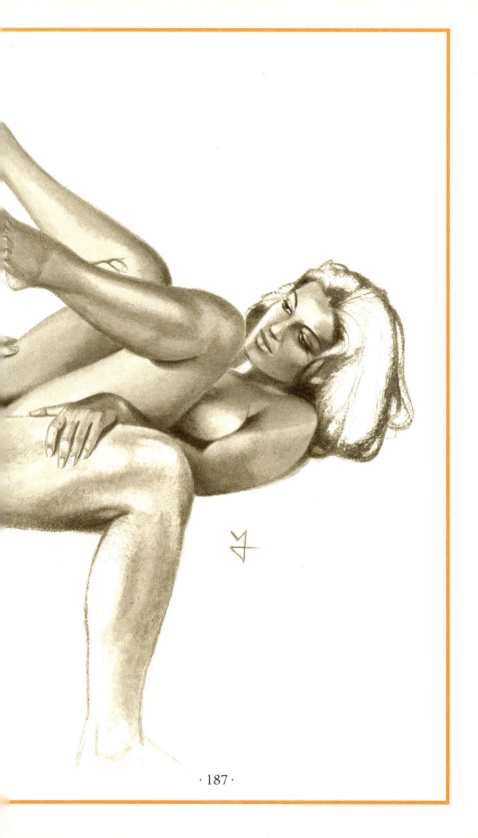

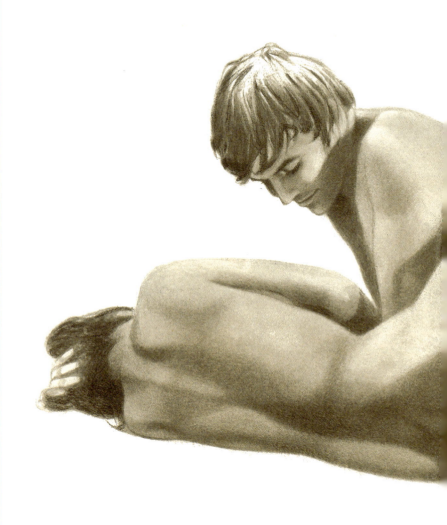

48 THE SCISSORS

The woman lies on her side with her legs apart and resting on the man's thighs as he penetrates her.

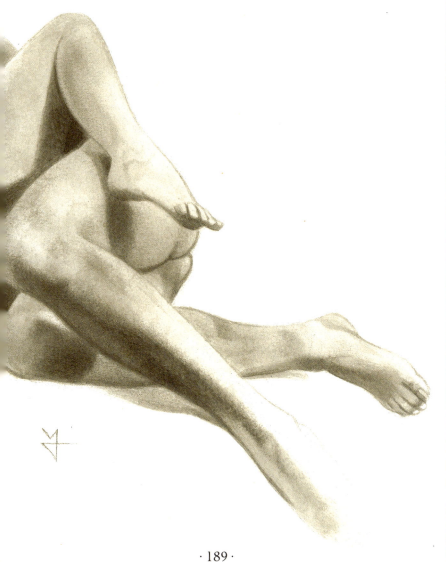

49 THE PASSING HAND

The man stretches out on his back, with his knees bent and his thighs apart. The woman lies on top, with her back to him, and impales herself on him as she supports herself with her arms. His hands are free to stroke her head and caress her breasts.

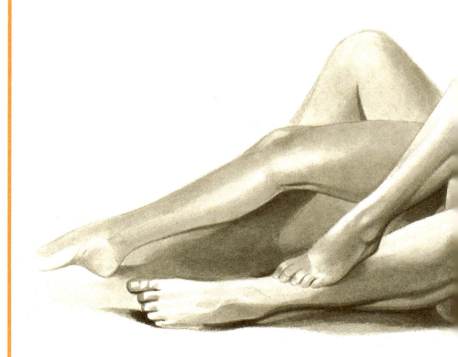

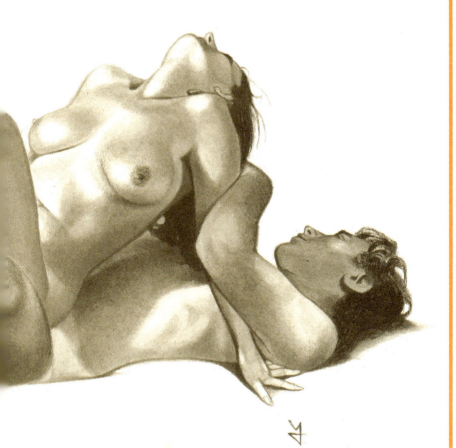

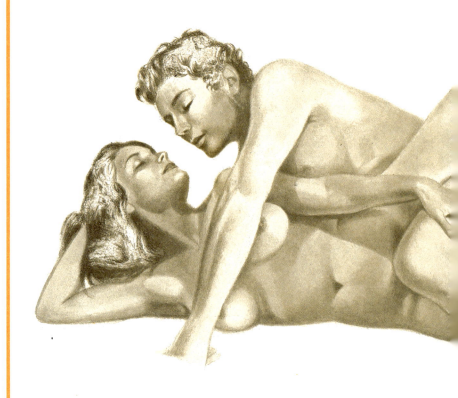

50 THE LAZY LOVE

The woman lies on her side, resting on her elbow. As their legs entwine, the man 'rides' her from behind. It is he who is responsible for all the movements. In this position, penetration is not very deep, but the sensations of bodily contact are very exciting.

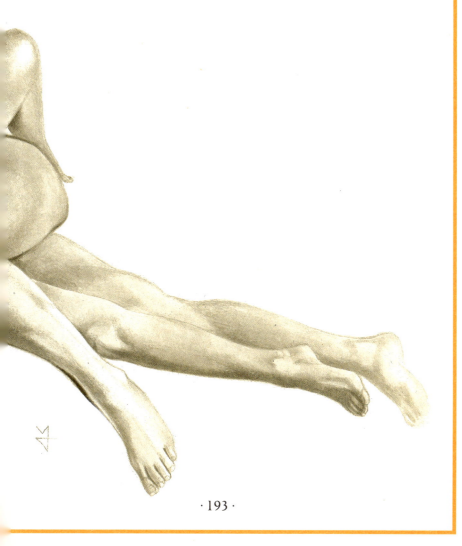

51 THE OPENING

Both partners kneel down, with the man behind the woman. He lifts up one leg. She does the same, resting her thigh on his. Penetration is deep, but this position cannot be maintained for long.

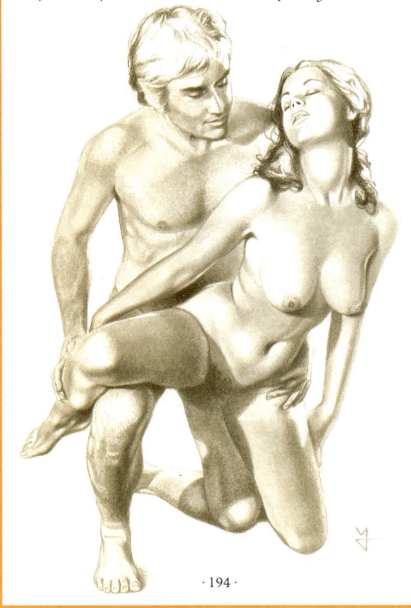

52 THE CONVERSATION

The man sits, supporting himself with his arms. The woman then sits on his thighs, 'riding' him face to face. This way she can caress his neck and ears – both very sensitive erogenous zones – and he, in turn, can kiss and lick her breasts by leaning forward.

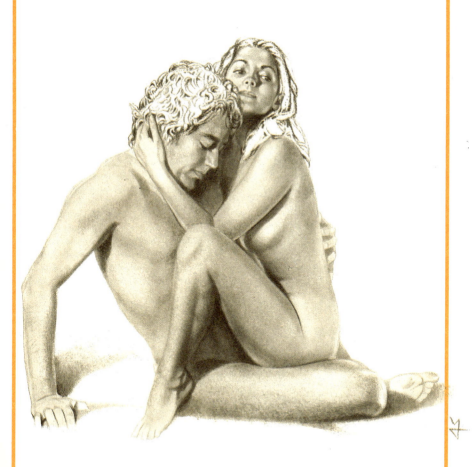

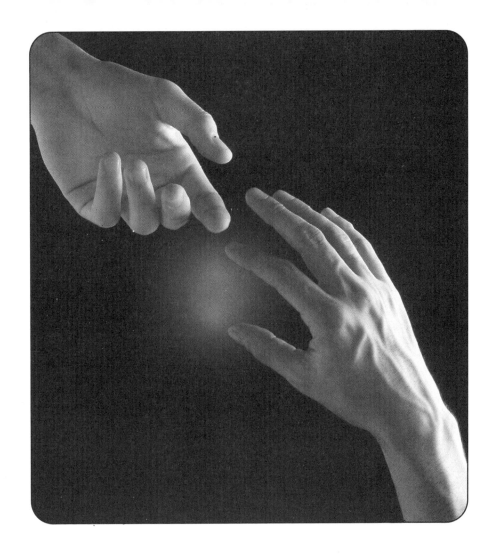

THE RISKS OF BREAK-UP

•

*The emotional and sexual problems
that line the path of a couple's life . . .
how one faces up to and resolves them.*

•

OPENING THE DIALOGUE

Even if sex education has made enormous strides, it is still limited to an explanation of the reproductive functions of the human body, without ever evoking the physical pleasure involved. Parents do not speak about it to their children and they, in their turn never – or rarely – dare to ask.

Thus a blanket of silence is placed over the whole question of sexuality and this continues right through to the time when young people reach the age of falling in love and having sex. They know how to express their affections but not their feelings and this can be the source of much dissatisfaction, which can end up by destabilising the couple.

"We have been married for more than a year," writes Oliver. "Julia was brought up in quite a strict family and used to controlling her actions and her feelings. We work in different places and so are very pleased when we meet up again in the evening. She really is a tender and happy young woman, who shows me her love in a thousand and one different ways . . . save the one of which I dream: to become engrossed in my pleasure when we make love, as I do in hers.

"I would love her to caress every part of my body, but I have to say that she is afraid to do it. She has never touched my penis. When I take her hand to put it on me, she pulls it away immediately, as if it is something dirty.

"However Julia certainly does not lack sensuality. Her whole body quivers in my arms when I take hold of her. I feel her desire and her pleasure, even though she never utters a word – not even the slightest sound – at such moments. I really suffer because of this and I do not know how to tell her without upsetting her."

Oliver's case is not exceptional. His young partner carries the burden of a strict upbringing, in which her parents' moral principles had forbidden all reference to sexuality. However she did have inside her a sensuality that her husband knew how to reawaken. But Julia has, for all that, still not been able to accept her husband's body or the pleasure that she feels.

Oliver must address the problem at an opportune moment, for example after they have made love, and explain that caressing a man's body is a natural action and that physical emotion can also be translated in words. To save their relationship, he must break the silence . . . with patience, with tenderness, with conviction. He has to make Julia understand that they could be even more happy together if their sex life was more balanced, more wholehearted.

Quite obviously, one cannot expect a miracle! Julia is not going to change overnight. Oliver must continue to bring up the conversation at the right time. Even if Julia protests and rebuffs him, arguing that she is very happy as she is, his words and phrases will gradually sink in and eventually she will have the courage to behave like the complete woman.

All sexologists confronted by such problems agree that sexual harmony relies on dialogue between spouses.

The success of any couple's relationship rests with effective communication and this habit must be adopted from the very start of their life together – talking together, having the courage to speak about everything, as much discussing the pleasure felt while making love as expressing one's reticence over certain caresses.

Certainly such exchanges of views are not always easy. We have been accustomed since childhood to say nothing of what we felt when we touched ourselves, never to mention genital organs . . . in short, to be ignorant – or pretend to be ignorant – of the existence of sex, a taboo subject in the majority of families.

"I was barely ten years old," recalls Mary, now in her thirties and married with three young children, "when my older sister Anne got engaged. I spent my time spying on the young couple, watching them kiss each other. One evening, when my mother came up to say goodnight, I told her that I had seen Anne and John making love. I got a good smack and was ordered never to speak about 'such things' again.

"In my innocence, I believed that what I had seen amounted to something really disgusting which had to remain secret . . . and for the next few years I continued to think that kissing on the mouth was actually making love.

"Some little while afterwards, when I was twelve, I had my first period. The sight of blood put me in a complete panic. My mother had not told me anything. (I found out a lot later that she thought I would not have my first period until I was fourteen, as had been the case both with her and my older sister.) I did not dare speak to my mother about what had happened, believing that too was in some way dirty. I cried all night. I was afraid I had a serious illness.

"Eventually I confided in my sister. She reassured me by explaining what had happened. Afterwards, I felt proud to have become a 'woman'. But for a long time I blamed my mother for having deliberately kept me ignorant of the 'facts of life'. That will not happen with my children, since I do not want them to suffer the anguish I went through."

The tale of Mary illustrates well the consequences of the attitudes of mothers who surround everything concerned with sex in a veil of mystery: the naivety of the little girl, which is excusable at her age, together with being confronted by a reprimanding mother, contributed not only to planting in her a false idea (to kiss is to make love), but also to preventing her from asking questions which, at the time of her first period, would have allowed her to understand what was going on inside her body.

This necessary opening of dialogue, which should start from infancy in the very bosom of the family, will then continue through to the life of couples living together. 'When people love each other, they should tell each other everything' must be the motto for those who want their union to succeed.

Amelia and Matthew both agreed to live together for a year before deciding on whether to get married. It was a kind of trial marriage. The two young people – nineteen and twenty-two respectively – had already had sexual relations but in conditions that did not seem to them very satisfactory: on the quiet, at their parents' place when they were away, in the woods, in the country, behind some rocks at the seaside . . . How they dreamed of making love in a bedroom behind closed curtains in a cosy bed.

The dream finally became reality in the form of a pleasant little bed-sitter, the principle item of furniture being a large bed – 'the place for all pleasures' was how Matthew described it to Amelia when they used it for the first time. There they played every love game imaginable, beginning with passionate caresses, adopting positions inspired by their mutual desire and culminating in ecstatic orgasms.

Then came the evening when Matthew took Amelia's head between his hands and drew it towards his hard penis, saying to her: "Take me in your mouth." Amelia was initially willing to try this erotic game but she very quickly felt a retching inside and pulled herself upright with tears in her eyes. Overcome with excitement, Matthew started insisting – even begging – to be given this pleasure, which he regarded as a token of his virility. Amelia was now crying openly. So he stopped and smothered her with kisses, asking her to forgive him.

Eventually she calmed down and succeeded in explaining the reason for her repugnance – the feeling that she experienced to be dominated and have to submit against her will. Matthew listened, then told her he did not mean to force her to do anything. He was simply reacting to an overwhelming desire. They fell asleep in each other's arms.

This frank discussion had re-established between them a climate of mutual trust that a hostile silence or obstinate sulking would without any doubt have completely destroyed.

In consequence, Matthew used more psychology, bearing in mind his girlfriend's reticence. For her part, Amelia understood that it was possible to love every bit of her loved one's body.

SHOWING MUTUAL RESPECT AND ACCEPTING DIFFERENCES

Differences in temperament and variations in mood are such that, even with a very close couple, the two partners can find themselves at odds with each other.

For example, one Sunday late in the afternoon Daniel wanted to make love and indicated this to his wife by caressing and touching her and whispering sweet words in her ear. But Fiona was not at all in the mood. She had a meal to prepare for some friends they had invited to dinner. She also had to dry her hair and get dressed. In short, she evaded the amorous and insistent suggestions from her husband, who then went and sulked in front of the television.

What can one do in this kind of situation? Should Fiona have accepted and made love when she really did not want to just to satisfy Daniel's desires?

In our opinion, with a couple, both partners must consider each other as equal and independent. The woman is under absolutely no obligation to be submissive, even if that was for many centuries her traditional role.

Without waving the feminist flag, Fiona should have been able to explain kindly to Daniel why she had to reject his advances, rather than saying to him: "It's all right for you. You've got nothing to do!"

A little marital tiff, you might say, and not serious. But it could lead to feelings of frustration and aggression if it was repeated for this or other reasons.

Differences of opinion over matters of sex do have more serious repercussions for a couple's harmony. One of the most frequent is the lack of agreement over the sexual needs of each partner. One feels the urge to make love three or four times a week, while the other finds that once is sufficient.

Let us look at another case where there was disagreement over the sexual needs of a couple married for three years.

Diane had a strong sexual urge and thoroughly enjoyed making love – so much so that she used to make advances towards her husband Lloyd every evening. The trouble was that he did not share her appetite for sex. Nevertheless, he forced himself to satisfy his wife, since he was afraid that she might accuse him of lacking virility.

Obviously the situation could not go on for ever, with Lloyd feeling obliged to make love more often than he naturally wanted to. He began to realise the horror of this fiasco. His self-esteem suffered badly and, to add to his misery, he had to put up with constant recriminations from his wife.

So how can one resolve this type of crisis? By analysing it together instead of trying to brush it under the carpet. By speaking openly, sincerely, honestly ... each one stating clearly their feelings without accusing the other.

Speaking about sex is not always easy, but the hardest part is starting. Once you have established some communication, you will feel such relief that you will be able to talk a lot more freely.

The aim of such discussions is to find some ground for conciliation. Both must commit themselves, obviously in all good faith, to join forces in order to find the best possible solution as far as sex is concerned. The success of such an exercise demands a lot of love, courage and a strong sense of joint responsibility.

There is no magic formula for complete success. But by showing mutual respect and an acceptance of existing differences between each other's sexual instincts is definitely the key to a lasting relationship.

KNOWING HOW TO TAKE THE INITIATIVE

"I am never satisfied. I am always hungry for love, hungry for the man I love, for the man I married three years ago. But he says that with a couple it is up to the man to take the initiative in these things."

Beatrice, who is twenty-four, is not the only one to know and have to live this problem – the frustrating attitude of a husband who wants to confine his wife to a passive role. Thirty-two-year-old Helen confides that after seven years of marriage her husband Ian is still not always happy when she solicits him to make love. The first step must come from him.

How should one react in such situations? Their origins are certainly ancient and traditional. The male is the master who makes all the decisions. While one would normally expect to work towards the sharing of responsibilities in one's married life, there still exists among numerous couples an imbalance to the detriment of the female.

Before the quality of one's emotional and sexual life deteriorates, it is necessary to start talking – without drama, without blame – and express one's feelings at the right moment, possibly by profiting from an intimate situation where one can have a real heart-to-heart. Women, incidentally, are much better at doing this than men.

One should not attack the subject directly. Far better to lead up to it gently, perhaps by making reference to the confidences of a friend or by using an example from a film or a television programme. By talking about the problems of others, one can then bring the discussion round to one's own situation.

Watch your partner's reactions and, if you feel they are particularly negative, return to the subject later. But, in order to be constructive, you must always speak with an open heart.

Love is not just a sentiment. It is also an action. And this should represent the second phase of one's attempt to reach perfect harmony. A little cuddling each evening, tender kisses, all done gently without any sexual aggression, should form part of one's everyday expression of love and sensuality and, as such, will provide the best way of arousing your partner's desire without appearing to demand it.

The testimony of Corinne, who is twenty-nine, is particularly revealing on this subject.

"In the house, each of us has our role. Martin does the DIY, the gardening and the heavy work, while I do the cooking and all the other chores. We pool our two salaries – no problem there. We share the same interests and leisure activities. In short, perfect equality . . . just as far as the bedroom door. There, I haven't even the right to speak. If I feel in an amorous mood, there's no question of showing it. I must wait on the pleasures of my husband.

"Or, rather, I had to wait on his pleasures. A year ago, all that changed. I made the most of a holiday, away from any problem of work, a dream beach, the complete relaxation. One night in a little Italian bistro, with the help of some Chianti, I said to Martin: 'I love it when you stroke me. I love it when you make love to me. I love touching you, feeling you against me.' And, under the table, I put my legs round his.

"We returned to the hotel. Since he was feeling very hot, I made him a luke-warm bath and I washed him all over. Then I dried him and didn't let him move a muscle to help. What followed after that incident was exactly what I was hoping for. Little by little, Martin got used to letting me take the initiative. Now, when I want, he responds to my advances just as I respond to his. We say very little when this happens, since our gestures are sufficient. And we are both happy... and equal."

Learning to communicate, to open oneself up and move towards one's partner together form one of the great secrets behind any couple's harmony.

JEALOUSY: LOVE'S POISON

Even at the tenderest age, children are jealous: of their mother's tenderness, of the birth of a brother or sister, of the family's pet dog. This shows, certainly without analysing it, a need for exclusive possession, linked with the fact that, as babies, they felt themselves abandoned by their mother when they weren't being breast or bottle-fed or when, even for very brief moments, they were left on their own.

Obviously such feelings are normally unfounded but nevertheless can create a sense of suffering which can continue through to adulthood and affect those close to them – and particularly loved ones.

Those of both sexes who endlessly cross-question their partners, insisting on knowing their every movement and how they spend each minute of their day, are not always thus displaying a genuine interest but a very real sense of jealousy. As a result, the husband turns into an inquisitor and the wife into a private detective. And such suspicion of one's partner amounts to a denial of the other's personality, to their transformation from a subject into an object.

Either one puts up with it – or one doesn't, as is most often the case, especially when jealousy becomes an obsession and is clearly not justified.

Neither the flirtatious female nor the seductive male is necessarily unfaithful. They are playing a game, whether it be to reassure themselves or to assert their authority or even to stir up some passion and feeling in those they really love. Often their provocative behaviour is nothing more than a pretence – and final realisation is rare.

But jealousy is always potentially a real poison, a lethal passion which gnaws away at the victim and can eventually destroy him or her. It has the power to drive people to the worst possible excesses and even crimes of passion, as one knows only too well by reading the headlines in the newspapers. Without necessarily reaching such dramatic levels, daily marital jealousy can eventually ruin a couple's life.

"Felix is a woman's man. By that I mean he loves their company, knows exactly what to say to flatter them, enjoys amusing them, brushing past them or kissing them under a thousand and one different pretexts. And he has the knack of throwing those casual looks, the real meaning of which certainly doesn't escape me! That's my husband.

"I try to be reasonable, to hide my jealousy, to tell myself that Felix likes playing the seducer because it's in his nature and that he doesn't go any further than a little bout of charm . . . I am convinced that he loves me, that I am the number one in his life. Nothing leads me to believe that he is deceiving me, but at the same time there is nothing to reassure me that he is not. I suffer in silence, day after day, never daring to put the question directly to him or, for that matter, trying to find out the truth."

This confession, from twenty-six-year-old Pauline, illustrates perfectly the case of the wife whose husband flirts openly in her presence. Is he looking to stir up her jealousy to convince himself that she loves him? Or is he quite simply being carried away by his natural gift as a charmer?

We would go for the latter hypothesis and would equally advise Pauline to use her jealousy in a positive way—by making it known to Felix what is in her mind, without actually accusing him of being unfaithful.

It is quite normal that she should be pricked with jealousy and feel a little suspicious. No woman, no wife, unless she were completely indifferent towards her husband, could remain an impassive spectator to such games of seduction. Some react with anger, others with a feeling of inferiority.

Pauline, who states that she is certain about Felix's love, is still only suffering from a mild bout of concern. And it is just that that she must explain to her husband. In addition, through her behaviour, she must impose her own personality and promote her own values and qualities.

Jenny's story is rather different.

"I have always considered jealousy as an absurd sentiment and was persuaded that I would never be a victim of it, being as sure of myself in my married life as I am in my professional life, where I run an important business. For eight years Lawrence and I had been perfectly happy, with a relationship based on a deep and reciprocated love. He used to admire me and always approved of my decisions.

"And then, when we returned from our last holiday, I sensed a subtle change in him. He started spending time away from the house and found it difficult to look me straight in the eye. It was clear his thoughts were elsewhere. At first, I believed it was due to problems at work or possibly something to do with his health that he didn't want to speak about to avoid worrying me. The uncertainty was driving me mad.

"But gradually my concern turned to suspicion. Deep down I feared he had a lover. I had to know, but I felt ashamed at the mere thought of having to search out the truth.

"Then, one day, I cracked. I went through his pockets. You can no doubt guess what happened. There were letters and photos and a notebook full of meetings, all of which left me in no doubt. There I was, a woman who always thought herself so strong, immune to the torment I had seen others go through. Now I was myself the victim of an unhealthy jealousy. I said nothing to Lawrence, but I spied on him incessantly, questioning him on what he did with his time, rifling through his briefcase, listening to his telephone conversations, smelling his clothes.

"I lost weight, I hardly slept and I was no longer able to play the role of the happy wife. I was riddled with jealousy and I was afraid. We ended up by having an unholy row, in which the only things I achieved were to attack Lawrence for having a mistress and to create an even wider gulf between us. In the end, we separated.

"Now, when I meet a man I like and who likes me, every attempt at an emotional or sensual relationship fails because I am permanently plagued with jealousy. And that's been going on for five years!"

For Jenny, who was in her own words 'so sure of herself both in her professional life and her married life', we offer this quote from Marcel Proust: "Jealousy is often only a disturbing impulse for tyranny applied to things we love."

Although undeserving of the unfair reference to tyranny, being used to having her own way, to leading, Jenny considered herself immune to all petty feelings such as jealousy. In fact, it is not her husband's infidelity that hurt her so much, but the fact of having demeaned herself by looking for proof.

This in itself was humiliating – and, in addition, the realisation that she was not the only one in her husband's life. Having been forced off her pedestal, she was engulfed in the worst of jealousies since she continued to suffer afterwards.

The only way Jenny can escape from her dilemma is to regain the self-confidence that she lost through this cruel experience. Our advice would be to consult a psychotherapist who could help her to understand that it is natural to be jealous when there is good reason to be so – which is true in her case – and to get rid of all the negative feelings that arose as a result.

The following testimony from Vanessa illustrates another aspect of jealousy:

"When I married Arnold, I had been widowed three years. So I had already had a man in my life – my first husband – and also, following that, two other relationships although neither were very serious. At twenty-seven, it is difficult for a young woman to live completely alone.

"Then I met Arnold. It was love at first sight for both of us, followed by marriage. It was perfect harmony. We were madly in love. In brief, total happiness. But now Arnold is in the process of changing – and in a way that worries me. He doesn't stop asking me about my first husband and my lovers. He questions me in the most minute detail about what we did together.

"This retrospective jealousy strikes me as unfair and annoys me. I really take exception to Arnold trying to make me talk about my past. And the worst of it is he seems to enjoy doing it."

To be jealous of a loved one's past is a painful game from which some men and women gain pleasure. Vanessa's second husband is one of them. If they want to know in the most intimate detail the relationships the other half had before their marriage, it is to visualise in their head the pleasure that person experienced through another, and equally, the pleasure that he or she gave. Such unbearable images feed Arnold's jealousy. He suffers and enjoys it at the same time.

This type of situation can only worsen and make life hell for a couple. Vanessa should refuse to join in this little game and, at the same time, reassure Arnold of the love she feels for him. After all, is not the fact that she married him the best proof of that?

If excessive jealousy quite quickly becomes insupportable, the total absence of jealousy can equally be felt by some people as a sign that the other half is not interested or does not love them. It is wrong, because each person has his or her own personality, temperament and character. Just as there are blondes and brunettes, there are the jealous and the non-jealous. Perhaps the latter should ponder on these few words from an old popular song: "A little jealousy arouses a happy love that sleeps."

INFIDELITY: WOUNDED LOVE

Infidelity doesn't just exist in bedroom farces. And if doors are slammed, it is anger and grief which provoke such violent reactions and not the need to conceal some lover or mistress in a cupboard or behind a curtain.

Today, of course, there is another side to infidelity. The real fear of catching AIDS has slowed down the activities of the wayward husband and also the wife searching for new experiences. However, extra-marital adventures still fascinate some men and women for different reasons, which we will now look at.

EMOTIONAL DISSATISFACTION

This motivation concerns women more than men, although the latter are by no means exempt.

Let us consider the archetypal 'indifferent' husband, buried in a book or newspaper or glued to the television, who absentmindedly kisses his wife, doesn't show any interest in how she has been spending her day, doesn't notice personal details like a change of hairstyle or, without passing any comment, devours his favourite meal that she has spent hours in the kitchen preparing.

No, this is not a caricature. Such men really do exist, although they can still be very much in love with their partner and will prove it in bed. But they do not seem to realise that a woman is a human being too, and sensitive to all life's little pains. She also looks to marriage for support, for a little admiration from time to time, for sexual satisfaction but also for other manifestations of love.

Some men possess the same kind of sensibility, even if they give the outward impression of being 'hard'. They too need attention, constant tenderness and companionship. One must listen to them, show an interest in their work . . . even their health. In brief, they like to be petted, pampered, loved . . . If the woman in their life does not treat them in such a way, they are going to look elsewhere for someone who will fill this emotional gap.

SEXUAL DISSATISFACTION

Unfortunately this kind of dissatisfaction can reveal itself from the very start of a sexual relationship between a couple and most often arises from such problems as premature ejaculation or difficulty in getting an erection for the man or lack of orgasm for the woman.

These are certainly matters on which one should seek consultation and such sexual malfunctions should normally be rectified with the appropriate treatment *(see Chapter 6)*.

However, when a couple experiences problems of sexual appetite, for example if the sexual urge comes twice a month for one and three times a week for another, then there is certainly a sexual dissatisfaction somewhere. Equally responsible for this condition is a marital weariness which can, after a number of years, affect a couple.

Love is always present, but the sexual enthusiasm becomes dulled. This is often the fault of having to search to renew previously successful techniques, of having to skimp the foreplay, of having forgotten the pleasure of the other for one's own benefit.

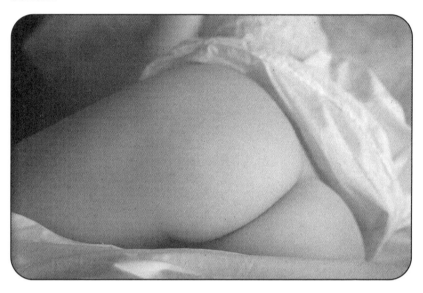

It is an insidious problem. One does not see it before it happens. And then, one day, whether it is the man or the woman, the true state of one's sex life becomes apparent. And this is the first step towards the occasional infidelity – or worse, a relationship with another person.

THE NEED TO PROVE ONE REALLY EXISTS

This is common among both men and women and can be the backcloth of the two previous motivations – emotional and sexual dissatisfaction. This source of infidelity involves those who feel themselves, rightly or wrongly, bullied in their professional life and to whom the family hardly gives any consideration.

As a result, one never asks for their advice and certainly never listens even when it is given. One feels as though one is living in a china shop.

Such people are ready to give themselves, body and soul, to anyone who will treat them as men or women with an important role to play in their life and with responsibilities to assume on their behalf.

THE WHIMS OF AGE

We all know the emotional problems that middle-age can cause. And do not think that it is just the men who are the victims. It happens to women, too.

Around fifty, some men and women (not all, of course) experience a sort of frenzy to live it up, whether this comes from a desire to catch up with lost time or to make the most of the final few years before they get too old. Their choice is most often young people, sometimes the same age as their own children, as they seek new amorous adventures.

These liaisons, struck up with the dual purpose of love and sex, are difficult to sustain and sooner or later deteriorate into a stormy relationship followed by the inevitable break-up, which leaves the victim scarred for a long time afterwards.

TAKING ADVANTAGE OF OTHERS

There is no shortage of people today who willingly profit from the weaknesses of others. Women who work are in daily contact with men and some will happily go along with any advances made to them. For their part, the men are only too pleased to put their hands in their pockets and spoil them. Equally they do not hesitate to tell the women they meet at work how pleasant they find them.

Such approaches often work. But it does not last. The women and men who create such opportunities and profit from them are only looking for a brief adventure – out of curiosity or simply to have an extra taste of pleasure. And it does not prevent them from going quietly back home in the evening to their husband or wife... and fantasizing about 'the other one' as they make love with their normal partner.

TIT FOR TAT

This popular expression illustrates the cases where the infidelity of one partner is balanced by the infidelity of the other. It is, if you like, a form of revenge, of getting one's own back, which leaves a bitter taste with the person who chooses to subscribe to such practice as a show of strength.

So these are the six causes of infidelity we encounter most frequently. There are others, of course, but it is impossible to class them in any particular category. These would include the state of one's health or a long period apart, for example.

SHOULD ONE ADMIT TO BEING UNFAITHFUL?

A delicate question, since so much depends on the personality of the individuals concerned, on the nature of the extra-marital relationship and on the continued existence of love between the couple.

As a general rule, the 'innocent' party does not find out directly about his or her misfortune from the other half. There are plenty of wagging tongues about to bring the news and it rarely happens that such affairs remain a secret forever.

Reaction to the news will vary according to one's personality: tears, recriminations, threats... One's self-respect is always wounded and the jealousy that is provoked leads to passionate and sometimes violent exchanges. The important thing is to make the point about the nature of the relationship. If it was just a passing fancy, it is possible that it will not have any lasting consequences or fatal repercussions as far as the couple's future is concerned.

As far as a well-established and potentially lasting liaison is concerned, the situation is quite different. Any promises of breaking up the affair are then often false and the very acceptance by the 'offended' partner is a recognition of guilt.

Those who find themselves confronted with such problems must consider the situation and its consequences seriously before coming to any decision. And it is essential that no decisions are made in the heat of the moment which run the risk of being regretted later, even very much later.

One potential consequence – divorce – represents an irreparable break-up, especially when there are children involved. Any wife who was financially dependent on her husband will have trouble retraining for a job (one of the reasons why every woman should be able to earn her own living!). As for the husband, he will lose some of the psychological comfort he used to enjoy in the family home, will be forced into unsettling changes of habit and, in addition, will have to pay maintenance to his former spouse. You may think these are rather mercenary considerations. But they do nevertheless affect one's everyday life.

Those who finish up by accepting the infidelity of their partner are more numerous than one might believe. And a lot eventually end up being rewarded for their tolerance by a return to a normal life together. It can take months, sometimes years. But it does happen.

"I have never been unfaithful to my wife. There's no point. I love her." Of course we have all heard these fine words from people justifying the success of their marriage. But have they got anything to do with reality? We have known couples who were deeply in love and for whom the odd affair did nothing to upset their relationship.

Finally, we should add that in our opinion, when facing infidelity, there is no difference between men and women. While Stendhal could write more than a hundred and fifty years ago that "the difference of infidelity between the two sexes is so real that a passionate wife can forgive, while a husband cannot", we believe today this difference no longer exists. Both husband and wife are capable of the same sufferance and the same love. It is these sentiments which count and not the sexes.

SOME TESTIMONIES

Alison (age 48)

"I work in a bank where my job is to deal with people who are looking to take out loans. For that, I have a small, quiet office. One afternoon a young girl came in, sat down and quite calmly said to me: 'You don't know me, but I know you very well. Your husband has spoken a lot about you. I have been his mistress for two years. He didn't have the courage to tell you himself, which is why I am here. I am twenty and wasn't even born when you and Gary got married. He still has a lot of affection for you, but it's me he loves now.'

"I was struck dumb by the young girl's quiet reassurance. With what she had told me, I felt as though I'd been stabbed in the heart. I tried desperately to control myself as I searched for something to say without revealing my distress. I didn't ask her any questions, although I desperately wanted to. I simply said that I would speak to my husband about it and showed her to the door.

"That evening, Gary tried to reassure me that it was only a passing affair, that I was the only woman in his life and that he would put a stop to it all the next day.

"I discovered later that he had done nothing of the sort. I hadn't tried to find out. It was the young girl who rang me to say that Gary was still seeing her and that he could no longer live without her.

"This hell lasted two years. Open discussion with my husband only led to more false promises. Ten times I was on the point of leaving him. But there were the children, two teenagers who might easily have been badly upset, particularly since they were at that critical school age where adverse exam results could have affected their future.

"And then one day those horrible phone calls ceased. Gary had never stopped showing me the greatest of affection and tenderness through those difficult years, but suddenly I felt a subtle change in his behaviour. He was much calmer and more peaceful. That was five years ago. We have never since brought up the subject of that painful period in our life."

Alison certainly showed a lot of dignity and selflessness in the way she handled the situation when she discovered that her husband was being unfaithful. This shows a truly strong character, well in control of herself and someone with a lot of love in her.

Perhaps Alison would have been able to ignore the telephone calls in which the third party had showed such complacency in detailing her relationship with her 'lover'. But there is no doubt she would have suffered more from knowing nothing than from being told in this way.

All's well that ends well. However, the hurt still exists, even if neither side brings up the subject of this personal drama ever again.

Jane (age 31)

"We had gone on an organised trip to spend the Christmas holidays in the West Indies. For Martin and I, who live in Leeds, it was a marvellous adventure. The sun, the sea, the flora . . . a real dream. We had a chalet on the edge of the lagoon. During the day we went on trips or relaxed on the beach. In the evening, there was dancing and music.

"During the holiday, we got together with two other couples in the group, people like us in their thirties. In the evening, when we were dancing, I found myself more and more in the arms of one of the two other men. His name was George. He made the most of the dancing and the subdued lighting to kiss my neck and stroke my hips. I was carried away by the alcohol, the atmosphere, the ambiance and the fact that I was on holiday, away from work, family and my normal life. I did nothing to stop his obvious advances.

"Martin prefered to play cards while we danced and therefore didn't notice anything. He didn't even see me go back with George one evening to his chalet.

"Every night after that we did the same, making the most of Martin's love of the cards and George's wife's passion for midnight bathing.

"I returned to Leeds full of wonderful memories, but closed the book as far as George was concerned. I have never seen him again. Martin knows nothing of my little adventure, but I often wonder how he would react if he did."

Everything depends on his nature. As far as pride is concerned, he would obviously be angry for quite some time. And he would also be very jealous. But since it was only a brief flirtation with no repercussions, it is probably better that Jane's husband knows nothing of the holiday romance.

Claudia (age 29)

"I never telephone Christopher when he is working away from home, which is often two or three days a week. He tells me in which hotel he is staying and he calls me at home early each morning. We have been married for eight years.

"But one evening his mother, an elderly lady, was suddenly taken seriously ill. So I rang the hotel as soon as possible. When I was transferred to his bedroom, a woman answered the phone. I hung up and rung again. This time I had my husband on the other end. I told him what had happened with his mother and he said he would be back as soon as possible the next day.

"When he got home I asked the burning question: 'Who was the woman in your room?'. Relaxed and smiling, he told me that it was a secretary who had come with some papers for him to sign.

"Was he telling the truth or lying? I had to know one way or the other. I realised it was disloyal, but I questioned the people he worked with and his best friend. I even telephoned the hotel under any pretext. I just had to know. I eventually found out that each week when he was away Christopher met up with a young woman who worked for the same company. I cried. I screamed with grief. And then I decided to sort it all out.

"I gave him the choice – her or me. Cynically he replied: 'Both!' I felt humiliated. But I couldn't and wouldn't shut my eyes to the situation. We didn't have any children, so I chose divorce. For that I paid dearly: two years of depression, emptiness and despair. But now I feel all right. I am almost cured of the love I used to feel for this man and have started to look to the future."

Claudia's decision to split up with her husband was certainly a wise one, even if she had to pay for it with some difficult years. Christopher's reactions are those of a profoundly egotistical man.

The enquiry Claudia launched in order to find out the truth showed her to be too possessive to accept a compromise. And divorce is a lot less dramatic for a couple without children. This young woman certainly considered carefully all aspects of the situation before making her decision, however painful that turned out to be.

Pauline (age 35)

"Why should I accept a husband who cheats me? Because he is by nature fickle and has only had brief affairs and not lasting ones? Because we have three young children and it is not worth destroying their family environment? Because I am 35 and less desirable than when I was 20? Because financially I depend entirely on my husband? What good reasons these are for staying where I am to eat my heart out with jealousy!"

This case is alas only too common among women who are cheated, yet nevertheless loved, where the presence of children and total financial dependence ties them to the unfaithful partner.

Pauline's rebellion is obviously legitimate. But what can she do? Wait for the children to grow up a bit more so she can go out and earn her own living? That means years more of patience and suffering. Shut her eyes and say nothing? She is too lively, too spontaneous to keep quiet and too jealous not to let rip with frequent recriminations.

Probably the only solution lies in a pact, whereby both agree that to continue living together there must be some reciprocal rules about each one's freedom. This means that Pauline too can have extra-marital adventures and her husband must accept them.

In effect this kind of arrangement often results in bringing the unfaithful husband back to his senses – and back to the house, so disagreeable does he find the idea of being cheated himself!

SEXUAL WEARINESS

One of the greatest enemies of harmony between a couple is routine. And here the real danger comes when sexual weariness starts to set in. This phenomenon has clearly little to do with the deep feelings that unite a couple. But it does apply particularly to sexual behaviour that lacks variety.

A lot of couples believe, wrongly, that there is a perfect sequence for making love. The man, in particular, often practises a sexual technique which, because it satisfies him, quickly becomes repetitive. If this 'perfect technique' can at the beginning satisfy his partner, the lack of surprise elements will, in the long term, generally and inevitably reduce the excitement and the pleasure.

The example of Nathalie is significant here.

"I am exasperated by my husband's attentions before we make love. He is very eager, attentive and thoughtful. Each time he feels in an amorous mood, he redoubles his attentions and goes out of his way to create the ideal ambiance, notably in preparing a foam bath which I used to love relaxing in.

"To begin with, this was fine. But, after two years, this foam bath routine is becoming so predictable that, instead of feeling excited by the thought of what will follow, I find this whole ritual particularly irritating. In fact, if he prepares one more foam bath for me I think I'll go mad."

How could such a situation have developed? Through lack of communication. While Nathalie found her husband's behaviour irritating, she did not dare talk about it for fear of upsetting him. Eventually, she ended up by telling him that their sex life seemed to lack a little fantasy. Several weeks later, thanks to some changes in their foreplay, the two rediscovered without much trouble their harmony and sexual satisfaction.

LOVE ON THE HOUR

Our life is ruled by the clock and we have too little time to devote to matters of love. In a family where, in addition to work commitments, one has to look after the children, prepare the meals, visit or invite friends and do all the domestic chores, it is hardly surprising that sex is pushed into the background.

Generally, the time to make love is late in the evening, when both individuals are tired and possibly preoccupied with what they have to do the next day. The result is that one or the other is not really in the mood for sex and so any love-making is rushed or simply avoided altogether.

The same situation can develop if sexual intercourse always takes place at the same time of the day, for example when one wakes up in the morning, or only under certain conditions, perhaps after a bath or shower. It does not need much thinking about for couples to avoid getting into whatever type of routine.

EXCITING EXPERIENCES

For most couples, the bedroom is the one place reserved for making love and all amorous activities are strictly confined to the bed. However, the pleasure to be gained from experimenting with different situations is practically unlimited and such experiences generally enhance the spontaneity and the excitement.

When love-making has to be adapted to a new environment (for example, the living room couch or floor), the partners are virtually obliged to discover new positions and sensations. The very thought that they could be disturbed in the middle of having sex also adds for some people a certain spice to their activities.

The change in surroundings can make all the difference, whether it happens spontaneously or is planned. Soft lights and music, comfortable cushions, something to nibble and to drink and logs crackling in the fireplace can do wonders for those who have fallen victim to sexual monotony.

SEX GAMES

Often the fear of not being at one's peak can prevent one or other partner from relaxing sufficiently and can also affect the excitement and eventual pleasure. After several fruitless attempts, negative thoughts accumulate and one would then not know how many more times one should try in the hope of experiencing completely successful and satisfying sexual intercourse, having repeatedly failed to achieve penetration or orgasm.

Exploring someone else's body provides enormous physical and emotional satisfaction and tension is generally eased when sexual relations are, from time to time, considered as a sensual game.

Most couples always make love in the same positions. The most common is that of the 'missionary', in which the woman stretches out on her back while the man lies face to face on top of her. Just by the fact that this position implies an element of submission on the part of the woman, it can after a while cause a sense of physical as well as emotional frustration.

But even the most stimulating positions can end up by losing their charm if they are repeated systematically, because the sequence of sensations becomes too predictable.

Where the two partners lack experience, the risk of sexual boredom is even greater. Deprived of a sufficient knowledge of the variety of positions possible, of the techniques and sensations which can be incorporated into the act of making love, the couple have to use even more imagination to discover new ways of finding mutual satisfaction.

Through fear, timidity or excessive modesty, the partners very often do not dare to try something new since they dread the thought of failure or disapproval. This lack of sexual courage can be the cause of much tension within a relationship due to the fact that the couple incessantly repeat the same gestures, which become less and less satisfying.

In a sexual relationship, it is particularly important that the two partners share sensations and emotions. By failing to express their needs, their preferences and eventually their dislikes, they are depriving themselves of the means of achieving mutual satisfaction. The situation can be sufficiently satisfying for a limited period. But, sooner or later, the partner who feels that his or her needs are not being fully met will lose interest in sex play.

WORKING TOO HARD

Those who work too hard are particularly at risk of becoming bored with sex. As a rule, they return home late after a back-breaking day, already thinking of the tasks that await them the following day. And that is when they have not brought work back to the house to do in the evening or over the weekend.

Where this happens, the other half gets the impression that he or she is becoming less and less important and their sexual relationship suffers as a result.

Those who feel neglected have the tendency to get their own back by refusing to have sex on the rare occasions it is offered. And so the relationship reaches the stage where any love-making is spasmodic and got over with quickly and, as a result, the couple's harmony is destroyed.

Sophie, a thirty-three-year-old secretary in a large company, gets to the office at half-past eight every morning and never leaves before half-past six in the evening. When she gets back, her two children are waiting for help with their homework.

Her husband Jim normally returns about seven o'clock, suffering from the effects of a hard day's work in the hospital where he works as a physiotherapist and the long journey home on roads packed with traffic.

Then there is dinner to prepare and telephone calls to the family and clothes to get ready for the morning... A thousand and one little things to worry about, whose need and often urgency add to the burden.

When Sophie and Jim finally get upstairs, with the meal eaten and the children in bed, they are completely shattered and fall asleep almost immediately, holding each other tightly together in a deep and warm embrace. Love is ever present, but the desire is completely overshadowed by exhaustion.

This is, of course, just one case among so many of the ill-effects of overworking. Can one escape from this problem?

No doubt, providing that this state of mind, which leads one to think that it will all be different tomorrow, does not become firmly fixed as a routine. And to ensure this is so, it is necessary for both partners, who obviously love each other, to organise within their lives – however busy, however complicated – some moments for themselves where they can rediscover the pleasures of love.

Does it really matter if the housework isn't done just for one evening? Or if the children spend the odd night with their grandparents or some friends, to whom one can offer the same facilities in return?

Certainly you should never feel guilty about stealing a little time for yourself. It is vital to remember that those moments when you can caress each other, express your sensuality and make love freely and openly provide the all-important basis on which to support your relationship as a couple.

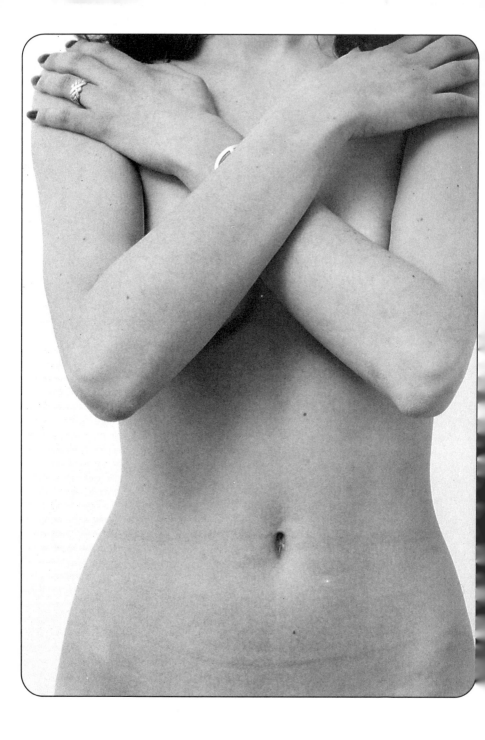

PLEASURE UNDER THREAT

·

*With men, as with women,
the sexual problems that endanger a relationship;
the organic or psychic malfunctions
that today one knows how to treat.*

·

OBSESSION WITH THE SIZE OF THE PENIS

"In my leisure time I practise my favourite sport – swimming. Obviously that means I end up in the changing rooms with other men. As we take our showers, I can see their penes and mine seems very small in comparison.

"I am twenty-two and in love with a girl who loves me too. We kiss and cuddle and get on very well together. But I do not dare go the whole way with her because I am afraid she will laugh at my small penis. It measures eight centimetres when relaxed. I fear that no woman can be satisfied with a penis of this size."

Jeremy's anxiety shows through in this testimony: fear of ridicule and also of not being sexually competent. And it is shared – wrongly, as we will see – by a large number of men.

We should make the point straight away that the size of the penis, at rest as in erection, varies from one individual to another. Within a few millimetres either way, the average length of a penis at rest is 8.5 to 10cm and its circumference 7.6 to 8.8cm.

According to the *Kinsey Report*, the average length of an erect penis varies as follows: 10.2 to 12.3cm – 12 per cent; 12.7 to 15cm – 20 per cent; 15.2 to 17.6cm – 45 per cent; 17.8 to 20cm – 20 per cent; 20.3cm and more – 3 per cent.

From inquiries and studies, notably those of the Americans Masters and Johnson, it is possible to confirm that the larger a penis measures when at rest, the less it increases in size when erect.

It is worth noting that the morphology of the individual can affect the size of the penis. For example, a tall, thin man often has a long penis, while someone who is considerably heavier than the average generally has a thicker but shorter penis.

Here are some statistics on the circumference of a penis when erect. A length of around 16cm corresponds to a circumference of 9 to 13.2cm; a length of 14cm corresponds to a circumference of 11.7 to 13.7cm; and a length of 17.5cm corresponds to a circumference of 12.4 to 14cm. These measurements were taken during a study of a hundred and twenty white males and can only therefore be considered as a sample and not definitive as examples of the absolute model.

It is difficult to get precise measurements when it is at rest, since it will vary in size depending on the blood circulation, the surrounding temperature and psychological tensions.

If you want to measure your penis, this is how you should do it. When the penis is erect, place your tape measure on top of it and measure from the pubic bone to the end. Take your measurement of the circumference about two centimetres from the gland.

VIRILITY IS NOT MEASURED IN CENTIMETRES

Sexologists the world over are absolutely in agreement on this subject: the size of the penis has nothing to do with the amount of pleasure given and felt. The psychological block suffered by plenty of men who think their penis is too small does not square up with the reality of a woman's anatomy.

The vagina measures 8 or 9cm long and, when excited, increases by about 2.5cm. Thus a penis of 10 to 12cm when erect will fill the vaginal cavity perfectly. And even if this is not the case, the partner would feel the pre-orgasmic and orgasmic pleasure, since only the first third of the vagina, from its opening, is sensitive.

On the other hand, the penetration of a penis that is 20cm or more in length can over-stretch the vaginal tissues and be painful for the woman.

"Let me tell you about my personal experience," writes thirty-two-year-old Serena. "Dominic was a handsome man, six foot tall, muscular and with a lot of charm. He possessed powers of seduction I just couldn't resist. After several evenings out, I finished up by agreeing to go back to his place. There he admitted to me his concern about the size of his penis – twenty-one centimetres when erect.

"That made me smile and I reassured him there was no problem. But when he entered me, I couldn't help crying out with pain. I felt that my vagina was being stretched to breaking point. It was unbearable. Dominic was already used to such reactions from his other girl friends. I didn't see him again.

"Now I am married – to Steven, whose penis of twelve centimetres when erect gives me the greatest orgasms possible."

We have numerous testimonies which prove the fact that there is no relation between the size of a penis and erotic superiority. Here, amongst others, are two letters on the subject.

Muriel (age 24)

"My husband has a penis which, when erect, measures nine-and-a-half centimetres. Before we first made love, he felt terribly worried, persuaded that he didn't have the ability to satisfy me. But we were very excited, very loving – and still are. When he entered me, I had a feeling of fullness in my vagina and his thrusts, sometimes quite violent, drove me to have a marvellous orgasm. We have been married for four years and I can assure you that there is no reason whatsoever for a man to depend on the size of his penis to give a woman sexual happiness."

Laura (age 20)

"I get lots of happiness from Harry's penis. When it's resting, it's as pretty as a baby bird in its nest. I take it in my hands and it swells up, though only to adolescent proportions. As I child, I did accidentally see my uncle's penis. It seemed so big, just like an animal's, and I still have terrifying memories of it. For many years I thought about a penis of that size entering me, going right through me, ripping me apart. I ran away from any sex. Then I got to know Harry, his tenderness, his softness . . . his penis. All my fears have gone and the man I love gives me infinite pleasure with his ten centimetre erect penis."

Alternative positions

These testimonies – and plenty of others along the same lines – prove that the quality of pleasure is not determined by the size of the penis. However men continue to argue over this subject, ignoring or wishing to ignore the fact that it is not the size of the penis that matters but more especially the way in which one uses it. Thus certain positions are more favourable for deep intromission than others.

For example, in the 'missionary' position, where the man lies stretched out on top of his partner, only two-thirds of the penis penetrates the vagina. But if the woman lifts up her legs and bends her knees, the penis can penetrate two or three centimetres more. It is the same when the woman straddles the man, keeping her back very straight.

The 'greyhound' position is equally recommended, where the woman kneels and opens her legs, supporting herself on her outstretched arms. If the man kneels behind his partner, he can introduce his penis to its full length into the vagina.

Exercises

There is another technique that allows the woman to feel the maximum benefit from the male organ: contracting the vaginal muscles in order to grip the partner's penis more firmly. The muscles in the vaginal opening and sheath are sphincters, just like those around the anus, and every woman can make them contract when she wants.

Those who do find difficulty in achieving this should practise doing it by sliding an object of roughly the same shape as a penis into the vaginal opening. About ten minutes of daily exercise will produce excellent results after just a few days. The woman can then user smaller and smaller objects, thus strengthening the muscles which will then contract in the same way around her partner's penis.

An American obstetrician Dr H Kepel made a study of the exercises required to strengthen the band of muscles around the vagina. These are very simple and can be practised anywhere anytime: while doing the washing at home, typing in the office, even when travelling on public transport.

The muscle that must do the work is that of the perineum. To find it, while you are urinating, make yourself stop suddenly several times. It is this muscle which is contracting.

Dr Kepel's exercise should be practised three times a day.

Exercise 1: Contract the muscle for three seconds, then release it for three seconds. Repeat this alternately, about ten times to begin with.

Exercise 2: Alternate between contracting and releasing the muscle ten times as quickly as possible.

Exercise 3: Contract the muscle and hold the contraction for three seconds. Then push as if you were going to stool, that too for three seconds. Alternate these for as long as possible, but not more than five minutes.

After a few days you should have achieved, in the course of the the different phases of the exercises, about three hundred voluntary daily contractions, which you will then be able to perform during sexual intercourse, thus gripping your partner's penis more tightly.

INCREASING THE SIZE OF THE PENIS

Such is the dream of all those who believe that their penis is too small. And the dream is further nourished by numerous advertisements for special creams, massages, developers of all kinds and miraculous methods inspired by Chinese and Japanese medicines.

Let us be quite clear about this. None of these 'miraculous remedies' work. And some even present dangers.

The ointments risk causing irritation on the sensitive skin of the penis.

The developers – glass tubes with a rubber pipe connected to a bulb – can create an illusion at the moment when they are used. The limp penis is inserted into the tube and a vacuum created by pumping the bulb. The penis stretches to its maximum erection. Unfortunately this stretching does not last. And if the glass happens to break, the consequences for the penis could be quite damaging.

The more serious sexologists have studied closely the various methods proposed. The conclusions they have drawn over such treatments are not favourable. In essence they have found them often expensive and always useless.

So, despair for the 'little penis'? Absolutely not. Sexual know-how and shared love brings for all couples the complete satisfaction, which is one of the strongest elements of life together.

PREMATURE EJACULATION: A SEXUAL PROBLEM THAT CAN BE CURED

For men who have this problem, it is the pride that suffers – and of course the love for their companion. As a result, the complete life of the couple can be destroyed through this 'shortcoming'.

SOME TESTIMONIES

Sebastian (age 24)

"I was nineteen when I succeeded in convincing Laura, the girl I had been going out with for two months, to come back to the flat with me while my parents were out. We settled ourselves down on the bed in my room and I started to caress her, pushing my advances quite far. She reacted as I had hoped she would and I felt that she had the same desires as myself.

"The only thing that worried me was the thought that my parents might return home earlier than expected. So I kept my ears pricked and jumped every time the lift stopped on our floor. I did everything to get our love-making done as quickly as possible and penetrated Laura, who was quite willing. But I had hardly started to get into my rhythm when I ejaculated.

"This was my first experience. The second was no better – in the back of the car, which was also very uncomfortable. Since then, I have never been able to control myself for more than a few seconds. I have even managed to come before intromission. I am now twenty-four and my sex life has been a continuous series of setbacks."

Derek (age 27)

"When we were married, Alice and I made love like mad things. Each time she had several orgasms and, for my part, I was able to last as long as was necessary for her pleasure. Then our little girl was born. The delivery was very difficult and the after-effects extremely painful, so much so that Alice did not want to have another child. Equally, she did not want to take the pill or wear the coil. So we had to use the withdrawal method as a means of contraception and I had to pull out as soon as I felt I was about to come.

"For Alice there was hardly any pleasure, since she was above all preoccupied with the fear that I would not withdraw in time. For my part, the sexual game had lost much of its attraction and I realised that I was ejaculating more and more quickly, as if I just wanted to get a thankless task over and done with."

Roland (age 29)

"I try really hard to think about something else – the money I owe the taxman, the problems I have at work, my car that needs replacing ... But there's nothing I can do ... I ejaculate the moment my penis is in contact with my wife's vagina. To begin with, she made some rather disagreeable comments. Now she shows me a coldness I find hard to cope with. I love her and I feel humiliated by the fact that I cannot give her the pleasure she expected from our marriage."

Thomas (age 23)

"My wife and I – we are both twenty-three – devote quite a long time to mutual caressing and we get a lot of pleasure from this without even going as far as orgasm. But when I enter Helen, hardly have I started the rhythmic motion when, without fail, I ejaculate. Naturally this leaves her unsatisfied. The situation has been going on for two years now and drives me to despair. It also drives my wife to despair. I am ashamed of myself and equally afraid that she will go and look elsewhere for what I can't give her."

Marion (age 31)

"Julian is a marvellous husband, soft and gentle and full of attention towards my well-being. We share the same tastes and we would be completely happy together if, when we made love, he could make the pleasure last. Alas, after barely a couple of minutes, he cannot contain himself and ejaculates. This is far too brief a time for me to reach orgasm."

David (age 25)

"I am at my wit's end. I no longer dare approach a girl. I have met with so many setbacks since the age of eighteen . . . And that from the very first time I made love. I ejaculate in a few seconds."

Causes

These few testimonies express the distress both of men and couples. It is the sad complaint of premature ejaculation. But let us immediately reassure the victims of this sexual problem: in all cases a cure is possible. We will come back to this, but first let us define premature ejaculation.

Sexologists consider it as such when it happens between thirty and ninety seconds after penetration. It involves between 20 and 25 per cent of men of all ages. And it is the most frequent reason for seeking consultation with a sexologist.

This consultation is indispensable for the cure, because only a doctor can diagnose the causes of premature ejaculation and prescribe the relevant treatment.

One must distinguish between two types of premature ejaculation – primary and secondary.

Primary: This happens from the first sexual encounters.

Secondary: This occurs after an indeterminable period of normal sex life.

Through questioning the patient and eventually the couple together, the doctor can determine the type of premature ejaculation.

The determining factors in this problem most often involve initial sexual experiences that are hurried, incomplete or made uncomfortable by the fear of being surprised and the practice of coitus interruptus (withdrawal before ejaculation).

In no event is premature ejaculation connected with the habit of masturbation.

THE TREATMENTS

We should repeat here that the choice of treatment rests with the doctor and underline the fact that the success of the therapy depends on the couple's complete collaboration.

Stop and Go

This is the method conceived by an American doctor, James Semans. The woman stimulates her partner's penis up to the moment when he feels he is about to ejaculate and stops. Then she starts again. In this way the subject goes through an apprenticeship in the art of controlling ejaculation.

He can also use this method of training when his partner is not there through manual masturbation, respecting of course the principle of 'stop' and 'go'.

Normally it is necessary to practise such 'exercises' for at least three months before perfecting one's control. The great advantage is that this treatment is carried out at absolutely no expense and does not necessarily have to involve the co-operation of one's partner.

Squeezing

The American sexologists Masters and Johnson obtained some positive and spectacular results from the treatment of premature ejaculation in their clinic in St Louis. The therapy they applied, which they called 'squeezing', was for the couple and not just the man.

Squeezing involves a restriction of the male sexual gland carried out by the female partner during exercises programmed by the sexologist organising the treatment.

In one instance, the woman is seated with her legs apart, leaning against some pillows. The man, lying on his back, stretches out between his companion's legs, with his own legs well apart and his knees raised. In this position, he presents his penis to his partner, thus provoking an erection. He then masturbates the crown of the gland between his index and middle fingers, with his thumb resting underneath his penis.

At the moment when he is about to ejaculate, his partner squeezes these three fingers, without changing their position, around the base of the gland. She maintains this pressure for three or four seconds, which has the instant effect of suppressing the man's need to ejaculate, while his erection drops by between 10 and 30 per cent.

His partner then recommences, alternating between masturbation and squeezing. This session should last between fifteen and twenty minutes.

These exercises, which should be repeated for two or three days, are designed to achieve total suppression of ejaculation, which normally results after masturbation.

In the second instance, the man is completely stretched out on his back. His partner kneels and sits astride him over his genital organs, with her hands resting on his shoulders. In this position, the man penetrates his partner, both staying motionless.

When the man feels that he is going to ejaculate, he warns his partner, who withdraws and starts squeezing his penis for two or three seconds. Then she repositions herself on top of him and lets him penetrate her once again.

It is important to observe the advice to remain motionless, since this allows the man to get used to – or reaccustom himself to – contact with the vagina.

This exercise should be repeated for several days, after which the man can start to make some movements while the woman remains absolutely still. This way, the couple should be able to last fifteen or twenty minutes without the man ejaculating.

During the subsequent stages, coitus should first be carried out in a side-on position, then in other positions.

Biofeedback

This is a relatively recent technique involving the electrical stimulation of the muscles controlling ejaculation just to the moment when the patient has identified them.

He should then be able to contract them himself, without the aid of electrical stimulation, and so learn to control his ejaculation.

Naturally this method has to be practised in a surgery specifically equipped for the job. Two half-hour sessions per week for about two months, followed by personal training of ten daily series of a hundred contractions of the pelvic muscles for three months, produce interesting results. The check rate is about 5 per cent.

Hypnosis and injections

Dr Gilbert Tordjman recently developed a new two-phase method of treating premature ejaculation.

Phase 1: Two sessions with the couple under medical hypnosis which principally enables them to counteract the man's anxiety provoked through his fear of sexual failure.

Phase 2: Six sessions of injections of Prostaglandine E1 spaced through one week, which will ensure an erection lasting about three hours. This space of time allows the couple, in progressive stages, to recognise the levels of intense excitement, to still the fear of early ejaculation and to ease the frustration of the female partner.

Medicines

Medicinal treatments are rarely effective. Most often they act to ease the anxiety or, as anti-depressants, they delay ejaculation but induce problems of erection and lower the sexual appetite. In the majority of cases, positive results only appear during the period of treatment. After this stops, the trouble reoccurs.

The different products in use – creams, pomades and sprays – anaesthetize the various critical areas of the penis. This kind of temporary anaesthetic does delay ejaculation but its effect is short-lived.

While such treatment does provide a limited solution, it is advisable to ask a doctor to prescribe a product that will not risk irritating the very sensitive area on which it is applied.

Finally, you should remember that such locally applied products are only palliatives and not real treatments for premature ejaculation.

DIFFICULTIES WITH ERECTION AND IMPOTENCE

Nothing affects a man so much, whatever his age, whatever the shortcomings of his virility. These problems bring on the fear of failure and can even be the source of a 'sexual breakdown'.

Erection is a physiological phenomenon which happens in the same way to every male.

When at rest, the penis is small, soft and wrinkled. So how does it become smooth and hard under the effect of stimulation, which can be auditory (a tone of voice, a whisper), visual (the sight of nudity, erotic images), tactile (bodily contact) and sometimes even olfactive (perfume, body odours)?

To answer this question, let us examine the anatomy of the penis. It contains three little balloons, two situated on the dorsal side (these are the cavities that run along the penis) and one on the ventral side (this is a spongy body, along which crosses the urethra, the tube through which the urine and sperm pass).

These three balloons are made up of small cells which swell up with blood under the effect of sexual desire. This blood is carried along very fine arteries. The venules inside the balloons receive the blood and close up through a system of sphincters which make them absolutely hermetic.

Thus, under the pressure of the trapped blood, the penis becomes smooth and hard and points upwards and forwards. This is the phenomenon of erection, which is always a reflex action and not ordered at will. And, even with young men, it is possible to have difficulties in achieving it.

An erection is a vascular phenomenon, the swelling and rigidity of the penis deriving from the rush of blood in the cavities. But it is also a reflex which has different points of departure: masturbation, erotic fantasies, contact, sight and hearing. This reflex can thus be disturbed by different elements: fear of not being 'in top condition' or of making the partner pregnant, worry brought on from everyday problems (money, family, work), lack of time . . .

"We bought our flat, invested all our savings in it and are now going to be in debt for several years. Of course, we are happy to own our own place. But there is one particular drawback and that concerns our sex life.

"I still feel the same excitement when my wife Mary and I touch each other. We caress and I waste no time in having a good erection. Then invariably I start to think about all the bills I've got to pay and all that we still need to complete our comfort. The result: my erection disappears. That drives me mad, because I start to wonder whether I am in the process of becoming impotent. And I'm only thirty!

"The connection between my sexual failure and my preoccupation with financial matters has not escaped me. But I cannot forget my problems over money. It has become an obsession!"

To this letter from John, we should add that of Lawrence, who is twenty-seven.

"We live in a modern block of flats, not particularly well built, whose walls are literally 'transparent' to noise. Our neighbour on the right, an elderly woman of seventy-five and almost completely deaf, always has her television on full volume. To our left we have a pack of bawling kids and parents who scream back at them.

"In the evening, when we get back from work, Jasmine and I are sufficiently busy getting supper ready, doing a thousand-and-one different household chores and watching a bit of television to divert our attention from all the noises around us. But when we go to bed – we are early risers so early sleepers, too – we have no other choice but to wear ear-plugs to ensure some peace and quiet.

"Feeling Jasmine's body against mine arouses me but now I can no longer see it through to the end. Several seconds after penetration, my penis loses its size and rigidity. Then a strange thought occurs to me. It seems that the absence of noise cuts me off from the outside world and I become a stranger in my own body.

"It's about eleven o'clock when our neighbours finally go to sleep. And I fall asleep as well. After a hard day's work, I no longer have the urge to make love."

These examples illustrate a sexual reality: the fragility of an erection. In the cases we have mentioned, we are looking at young men in good health, who live a clean life without such excesses as tobacco or alcohol.

Problems over erection are due to physical causes and you cannot get rid of them just by the wave of a magic wand. Of course, if only John could win the national lottery to dispel all his worries over money or Lawrence and Jasmine could jump on to a magic carpet and fly off to an isolated country cottage where only the sound of birds singing would break the silence . . .

So what is the solution?

First of all, you should not let such situations become established or get engulfed in the logic of failure. Once, twice, three or even four times . . . That happens and you should not panic over it. But after that, it is essential that you face up to the problem, look for the causes and analyse them. Already, the fact that you are aware of this is a big step towards a return to normality.

Next, you should talk with your partner who, having been made fully aware of these problems of erection, will be reassured by the fact that you have not only acknowledged the situation but that you also have the desire to find a way out of it.

And finally, you should develop your love-making techniques, prolong the foreplay in such a way as to reach a state of extreme excitement which you can feed with your favourite fantasies – a little bit of mental cinema where, according to your partner's tastes, you can share the scenario with her or keep it for yourself. This is a good way of keeping up the sexual tonus.

It is rare for men not to have any fantasies and it is not necessarily a question of putting them into practice. In the majority of cases, it is sufficient just to imagine them.

Another important point. Concentrate hard on your partner, the softness of her skin, the smell of her body . . . Take in these sensations and adopt a completely open attitude towards sensuality, towards the animal instinct that sleeps in each of us.

More preoccupying and more serious than the temporary difficulties over erection is the 'repeated incapacity to maintain a sufficiently rigid erection for assuming or fulfilling penetration'. This is Dr Henry Dermange's precise definition of impotence.

Any man who knows about such problems of erection must seek advice without delay, before he gets a permanent feeling of failure in his head which could equally have an effect in areas other than just his sexuality. Through questioning and various medical examinations and laboratory tests, a doctor will be able to establish a diagnosis and, equally, the appropriate treatment.

It is important to distinguish between primary impotence, which occurs right from the start of one's sex life, and secondary impotence, which can happen after an indefinable period of a satisfactory sex life. In both cases, the search for the causes is essential.

Psychological: depression, psychological trauma, low self-esteem.

Medicinal: diuretics, antidepressants, neuroleptics, tranquillizers, slimming pills, anti-cholesterol drugs, all of which can cause serious difficulties with erection.

Endocrinal: insufficient amount of the male hormone testosterone.

Toxic: abuse of tobacco, alcohol, drugs.

One can more simply classify the causes of impotence as psychological and physiological.

Age equally comes into the reckoning. Masters and Johnson observed the sexual reactions of men over sixty. In comparison with a young subject, where erection was reached in between three and five seconds, this time doubled or even trebled with the older subjects. The force of the ejaculation reduced by a half. And, after ejaculation, the detumescence of the penis was immediate.

Of course this does not amount to impotence. The only problem here is that a man who is barely satisfied by his sexual performances – and whose partner is unaware of or wants to ignore his erotic needs – runs the risk of suffering from secondary impotence.

Now, age in itself does not cause either the desire or the possibility of sexual intercourse to disappear – and this well beyond seventy and even eighty. Naturally this depends on living a healthy life, paying attention to one's medical condition and not giving up the practice of sex, which is the best way of maintaining the possibility of erection.

In cases of real impotence, one will have recourse to appropriate treatments, prescribed by one's doctor. One should certainly not seek 'wild' remedies such as aphrodisiacs and various stimulants, which have absolutely no curing powers and, on the contrary, can have unfortunate side-effects.

It is important to repeat here that it is the doctor who should intervene and, if he or she judges it necessary, direct the patient towards a urologist, with the possible opportunity for microsurgery or implants in the penis.

SEX THERAPY

This method of treatment is based on the work of Masters and Johnson, where the two therapists provided guidance to couples, where the man was having erection difficulties.

The patient and his partner must learn that they are equal in the sexual domain and that the man can, without losing his dignity, accept the feelings of pleasure and above all be happy to play a passive role.

The cure begins with a re-education of erection. The partner stimulates the secondary erogenous zones through touching the penis. If erection occurs and then disappears, the man must feel absolutely no sense of failure. On the contrary, he must accept that he has no physiological problem. The presence of an erection, however fragile, is proof of that.

For the next stage, the partner stimulates the penis manually or orally right up to the moment when her companion reaches maximum excitement. This can diminish again. But if the fear of failure has been removed, the man understands that his erection will come back.

Penetration is only allowed when the man has regained complete confidence in himself. Coitus then takes place with the man in a stretched-out position. Following that, the couple will be able to adopt the following positions, face to face with the woman straddling her partner:

- The woman squats on the man, turning her back on him.
- The man and the woman lie on their sides, she with her knees bent and pulled up to her chest while he penetrates her from behind.

During these penetrations, the movements must be very measured. The coital to-and-fro will only take place after the end of the treatment. The therapy lasts about three weeks and will be started again, for a shorter period, in case of relapse.

This brief description simply highlights what is a complex treatment, which can only succeed if there is strict collaboration between the therapists and the couple – and, equally, between the two partners themselves.

SOME TESTIMONIES

John (age 32)

"Annabel and I have been married for almost ten years. We get on well together and our love is still very much alive. Three years ago, we had a very unhappy experience when our little boy Giles fell victim to a fatal illness. It was a terrible shock for both of us. But while she has had the will-power to pull herself together, I have allowed myself to become really depressed. I no longer have the desire to do anything, just to see my dear Giles again. At the same time I began to have problems with erection. And I wasn't even thirty! It is still no better and I feel ashamed of myself in front of my wife."

This confidence certainly calls for comment. Here we are faced with a case of secondary impotence, since John had experienced a normal sex life before the dramatic death of his child. A state of depression often leads to difficulties or even the impossibility of erection. So what can be done?

For a start, he must seek advice straight away. The difficulties he is experiencing are certainly not irreversible. A doctor will help him, first by treating his depression with medicines that will not endanger his sexual health. Then, free of anxiety and shame (it is John himself who uses this word) and supported by his wife's understanding and love, he will regain his virility.

Roger (age 59)

"I never thought that it would happen to someone like me, who from the age of nineteen has made love several times a week, with much pleasure not only for myself but also for my partners. And now it is finished! The desire is still there, but fulfilment is impossible. My wife has tried everything to excite me and I have dreamed up the maddest of fantasies. But my penis remains lamentably limp. Yet I am in good health, apart only from a little cholesterol problem over the last couple of years, for which I take some medicine prescribed by my doctor."

The cause of Roger's problems is probably the cholesterol or, more likely, the medicine he is taking to treat it. The majority of anti-cholesterol drugs have a habit of provoking trouble in erection and this unfavourable side-effect only comes after a few months. Happily not all anti-cholesterol drugs act in such a disastrous way. His doctor can change the treatment.

Luke (age 27)

"While other men of my age are in full possession of their virility, I am impotent. In fact, I always have been. I have never had a real erection when I have been with a partner. Sometimes I come when I masturbate. I don't dare go and see a doctor."

He must do so. And urgently! This situation is not going to resolve itself on its own. He needs to get it diagnosed. And the causes of his impotence need to be known so that it can be treated.

In such a case, the doctor will interview the patient at length and will no doubt make him undergo various tests, such as taking hormone samples to show whether there is a male hormone deficiency, evaluating the quality of the blood flow in the penis and using plethysmography (a technique for measuring the degree of erection) to identify the type of impotence, whether organic or psychic.

It is only following the results of such tests that the doctor will prescribe appropriate treatments.

Ralph (age 66)

"Towards the age of sixty, I started having erection trouble. I wasn't unhappy about it, nor did I feel humiliated, and my wife Yvonne seemed to have less need for sex than when we were younger. Then she fell very seriously ill and the time for making love had gone.

"Three years ago, I became a widower. I found it difficult to put up with the solitude after thirty-eight years of marriage to the woman I loved. Eventually I had the good fortune when visiting some friends to meet a woman whom I took to immediately. Since we were both independent, we decided to live together for a few months before getting married.

"And then my hell began! I really fancied Josie – but no erection. I was desperate, particularly since she was twenty years my junior and had a wonderful sexual vitality. I read in a magazine that a man could regain his potential through a penis support. I am ready to try anything."

It is not abnormal to have difficulties with erection when one gets on in years. According to the *Kinsey Report*, 25 per cent of men aged sixty-five see their performance diminish. But even at this stage in life, it is possible to have treatment and obtain satisfying results – and by means other than the one envisaged here, which is carried out in extreme cases.

It does, in effect, involve a serious surgical operation. This consists of introducing plastic rods into the penis which keep it permanently erect. A supple section at the base allows the penis to be folded back against the groin and thus to hide the erection inside one's clothes. Other types of prosthesis are also used. Quite clearly the choice here rests with the surgeon.

One should, of course, seek professional advice first since there are perhaps solutions other than surgery.

Leonard (age 67)

"I have heard about injections in the penis which enable older men to rediscover the virility of their youth. I no longer have erections."

This treatment does indeed exist. It involves injecting into the penis Papaverine, a vaso-dilator which after about ten minutes causes an erection that can last from between half-an-hour and three hours.

These injections, which are carried out using very thin needles, are painless. But the erection can continue after the time expected. Such an accident, which fortunately is extremely rare, needs to be treated urgently since such a state of 'over-run' erection, called priapism, can lead to permanent impotence.

THE PREMENSTRUAL SYNDROME: 77 PER CENT OF WOMEN SUFFER FROM IT

Plenty of women (about 77 per cent according to a recent survey by the International Health Foundation) suffer from various upsets before their periods, although few would associate them with the premenstrual syndrome, as do doctors and more especially gynaecologists. And this syndrome has particular repercussions with respect to the life of a couple, as much through physiological as psychological manifestations.

In the majority of cases, the upsets start several days before the period, growing in intensity right up to that moment and disappearing as soon as it arrives. Thus a woman can be quite unsettled for eight to ten days each month.

Tired, nervous and irritable, she becomes aggressive to those around her and more particularly to her husband. She feels poorly, suffering for example from headaches, flatulence and painful tension in the breasts, which accentuate her state of tiredness and upset her activities, whether at home, with friends or at work. It can also be that she puts on weight.

And finally her sexual appetite – libido – is affected by the premenstrual syndrome, whether it drops or disappears altogether or, on the contrary, makes matters worse.

We have seen that 77 per cent of women find themselves, from puberty to menopause, confronted with this problem and for 38 per cent it happens regularly each month.

SOME TESTIMONIES

Stephanie (age 37)

"Ever since I was thirteen – when I had my first periods – I have had to put up with ten difficult, not to say unbearable, days before the flux arrives to relieve me of my misery. I suffer from stomach pains, sometimes acute, as if I was being stabbed with a knife. My back feels strained and my breasts are so swollen and sensitive that I have real trouble putting on my bra.

"My mother told me it would pass when I got married. But this has changed nothing. Then she told me that giving birth would relieve me of my pains. I have had two children and I continue suffering each month."

Fiona (age 31)

"For a few days before my periods, my character changes and, sadly, not for the better. I am quite frankly odious, grumbly and aggressive. My husband is philosophical about my bad tempers. He has over the years learned that each month I go through a difficult period during which the demands of my feminine physiology make me lose all self-control.

"My ten-year-old daughter, on the other hand, cannot understand why on certain days I have absolutely no patience with her, to the extent that sometimes I even smack her unjustly. Then I feel guilty and swear never to do it again ... But, the following month, I am again caught up in the same stormy spiral."

Anne (age 24)

"Married for four years, Max and I make a happy couple. Our good humour is based on a perfect mutual understanding of all aspects of everyday life. Our love-making – on average, twice a week – is totally satisfying and I particularly appreciate those moments of real tenderness just before and after we have sex.

"So no problem, you would think. But yes, there is a problem. During the few days before my period, I become a different woman. I am in some kind of way dominated by desire. I need to make love a lot more often than usual. And it's for the sake of sex rather than pleasure. My attitude surprises Max, but he doesn't complain. Then, after my period, I become my normal self again. I don't have this fever inside me any more."

Other examples

There are plenty of other testimonies that provide evidence of the manifestations of the premenstrual syndrome: Felicity putting on five pounds in weight, Emma making too many mistakes at work, Margaret bursting into tears, Gina suffering from migraines which confine her to her room with the curtains drawn ...

To this black picture one can add insomnia, palpitations, nausea, hot flushes ... as many of the sicknesses women have for too long suffered in silence. Today they can and must react.

The premenstrual syndrome is a reality both studied and recognised by doctors who know how to ease it and often to cure it. You should therefore consult your gynaecologist who will advise you on how to live through these difficult days more easily and comfortably and prescribe a treatment specially adapted to your situation – for example hormones, vitamins and mineral salts.

THE PROBLEMS OF ORGASM FOR A WOMAN

DYSPAREUNIA: PAIN AND NOT PLEASURE

When the penis penetrates the vagina and the woman gets a feeling of pain, this is a sexual disorder known as dyspareunia. Anyone with this complaint should consult a gynaecologist without delay. There is no question of suffering the pain in silence, since it could become a serious problem in the relationship between a couple and lead to a halt in sexual intercourse.

There are two types of dyspareunia – superficial and deep.

Superficial dyspareunia: This is characterised by a pain coming just after the penis passes the vulva. The cause of this is most often a vaginal infection which today can be treated effectively. It can also result from a hymen that is too narrow. A light excision will open it. The operation is done in a few minutes under general anaesthetic. More rarely one can find a vaginal malformation.

Deep dyspareunia: The symptom of this is a pain at the back of the vagina during intercourse. The cause is most often organic: the presence of an ovarian cyst (which can be removed with surgery), salpingitis (an infection of the tubes which requires special long-term treatment) or endometriosis (the presence of small pieces of tissue which overlay the inside of the uterus on the neighbouring organs). In this case, the doctor will prescribe some high-dosage hormonal medication.

An examination by a gynaecologist will establish the diagnosis and from that the treatment of the cause. If the doctor has not diagnosed organic causes, it will be necessary to look for psychological causes of this sexual problem.

Often one finds a puritan upbringing at the source of the trouble, a rejection of all things to do with sex considered as dirty and the burden of being forbidden to touch or to masturbate. Here the woman can feel a sense of fear and guilt when she makes love.

VAGINISMUS: REFUSING TO MAKE LOVE

This is an involuntary contraction of the perivaginal muscles, which makes not only penetration impossible but also a gynaecological examination or simply the placing of a tampax.

Vaginismus most often results from psychological blockages: an upbringing of being made to feel guilty, immaturity, failure with the first attempts at making love. However, if someone suffering from this denies her partner's penis entry through inpenetrable spasms of all the pelvic muscles, she can gain some pleasure and even orgasm from appropriate caressing.

How can vaginismus be treated?

The doctor has to enquire fully into the patient's background over several sessions before conducting a clinical examination, which as we have mentioned is difficult since the vagina will close up at the slightest touch. This is to confirm that there is no organic cause of the problem. Having established there is not – and this is the most frequent result – the patient will have to undergo a sexual reconditioning.

Relaxation is the basis of the treatment, which is completed with practical exercises by the woman alone or the couple together. In essence, the vagina has to be progressively 'tamed' in gentle stages using a finger. Masturbation is part of these exercises. But there is absolutely no attempt at sexual intercourse during the period of treatment.

FRIGIDITY: LITTLE OR NO PLEASURE

Frigidity – or anaphrodisia, to use the medical term – is the absence of excitement and satisfaction in the woman during coitus or, quite simply, the lack of desire or sexual pleasure.

Nowadays, we make the distinction between frigidity, as just described, and anorgasmia, which is the total lack of awareness of orgasm.

Frigidity and anorgasmia

For many years, notably in the Victorian age, under the influence of puritan values, sexual intercourse among married couples had only to be procreative. Pleasure was considered as diabolical and shameful, for the woman at least. For their part, the men could not deny the pleasure that accompanied orgasm, since ejaculation carried the proof.

The woman nevertheless had the obligation to submit herself to her 'conjugal duty' to relieve the sexual tension of her husband who otherwise had recourse to the services of prostitutes to fulfil his fantasies.

A hundred years ago, sexual repression forbid all expression of sexuality outside of marriage and procreation. Masturbation was considered as a disease which made one deaf, caused hair to fall out and led to madness.

It was difficult for Freud, without any other observations but the evidence from his patients, to measure the orgasm of the female, whom he called elsewhere 'the black ⟨...⟩ was consequently virtually impossible for him to env⟨...⟩ woman did not find pleasure, as the man did, desp⟨...⟩ procreative standpoint over coitus.

To satisfy the intolerant attitudes of his time, he p⟨..⟩ the view that, with a woman, there were two sorts of orgasm: the one, puerile, came through masturbation; the other, adult, came through penetration. He conceded, however, that the two functions of pleasure and procreation 'did not always totally coincide'.

Nevertheless, it was established that the woman could, like the man, experience pleasure and orgasm by rubbing her genital organs.

A quarter of a century before Masters and Johnson, with the help of progress and the minute scientific detail of a collection of Americans, measured the feminine orgasm, a Dutch gynaecologist Theodor Van de Velde, author of the book *The Perfect Marriage*, considered the genital kiss – cunnilingus – as 'particularly suited to arousing the sensuality of frigid and inexperienced woman'.

At a time when cunnilingus and fellatio were reproached as perversions, he did not hesitate to confirm that 'the genital kiss is perfectly legitimate, moral, aesthetic and hygienic'.

He wrote: "Coitus, just as nature wants it, makes the woman undergo vaginal and clitoral excitement combined . . .", but he advised that nature should be helped by accompanying the vaginal penetration with clitoral stimulation using a finger. This method is still recommended to enable a 'frigid' woman to achieve orgasm during coitus.

Van de Velde attached extreme importance to foreplay, which provokes excitement in the woman and induces vaginal lubrication, thus facilitating penetration. With good reason he regarded 'games of excitement' as necessary for provoking in the woman the 'erotic feeling', the desire and the facility to be penetrated.

He added that, if the erotic feeling was lacking, "whoever then, despite everything, practises coitus is behaving like a brute and an egoist, because he will leave his partner unsatisfied."

Certainly, Van de Velde was mistaken on a number of points. But equally some of his advice, such as that mentioned here, is still used today in the sexological treatment of frigidity.

While, however, his work had enormous repercussions at the time, the publication of the research by Masters and Johnson completely overshadowed it. Of course, their research benefitted from three major advantages: technology, the move towards a new liberalism and the development of the media.

With the support of measuring devices, Masters and Johnson

thus able to define the female orgasm: a series of involuntary contractions of the pelvic floor, from three to fifteen according to the level of excitement and at 0.8 second intervals. Therefore the orgasm does not last more than twelve seconds.

Their great revelation that there was but one orgasm went a long way to relieve women's uncertainties and inhibitions. Whatever the origin of excitement – whether physical through stimulation of the clitoris, vagina or breasts, or psychological through fantasies from reading or viewing erotic films – orgasm happens in the same way, through a variable number of contractions of the pelvic platform.

They concluded that the essential for a woman was not the method of stimulation used but the possibility of achieving orgasm. Despite the proliferation of sexual information over the last twenty years or so, this has not been accepted without resistance and still seems to be overlooked.

"Having lived with Francis for two years, I was concerned that I felt strictly nothing when he made love to me. I became even more worried when I started spurning his advances, which did nothing for me, and his embraces, which annoyed me more than anything. My love for Francis was dwindling. So I decided to go and see a doctor and, despite my embarrassment, to tell him about the problem – something I had never done with my husband.

"When I confessed to him that I was frigid, his only response was: 'Take a lover'. I was horrified. He didn't seem in the least bit interested in the sexual relationship I had with my husband. He hadn't looked further to find out if I knew what orgasm was like. In fact, I did. I had been masturbating since I was twelve. But I felt nothing of this kind when Francis penetrated me and I remained persuaded that it was just in this way that I had to experience it.

"A few months later I ended up following the doctor's advice and found a lover. He embraced me and then penetrated me and carried on so long that I began to choke. And still I felt nothing. I found another lover. And then I understood. He really loved caressing and searched to give me pleasure before thinking of himself. He could spend a whole hour kissing my breasts and my vagina and running his fingers all over my body. Like this, I had already had several orgasms before he decided to penetrate me. I was in such a state of excitement that, when I felt the contractions of his penis as he ejaculated, I had another orgasm.

"In a single moment I discovered, along with the pleasure, plenty of interest in sexual relations and I learned a lot at the same time."

This example of Mary, who is thirty-eight, reveals some interesting facts:

* Ignorance of a woman's reactions within a couple can be a disturbing element in the stability of the relationship.
* The woman can obtain sexual satisfaction other than through penetration.
* Realising orgasm through masturbation enables the woman to realise it when the sexual contact is well-directed.

The notion of anorgasmia comes in here. Can one describe as anorgasmic the woman who, having never masturbated, is totally ignorant about orgasms and only knows of them through description in books of fantasies?

All the treatments carried out today, following the work of Masters and Johnson, aim to make the anorgasmic woman aware of the reactions in her body, to make her discover orgasm. The most recent and, without doubt, the least demanding is the laser treatment pioneered by Dr Jacques Waynberg.

It consists of two phases:

* The application of a moderate laser beam on the genital parts, the heat of which provokes a flow of blood similar to that produced in the phase of sexual excitement.
* Masturbation training for the woman to provoke naturally the congestion of blood that leads to orgasm.

When through this method – or others that have also proved successful – the woman who knew nothing about the orgasmic reflex achieves it, anorgasmia stops. And the woman who, through whatever process, realises orgasm is not frigid.

So, any concern about the absence of vaginal satisfaction – as much for the woman as for the man – is a myth.

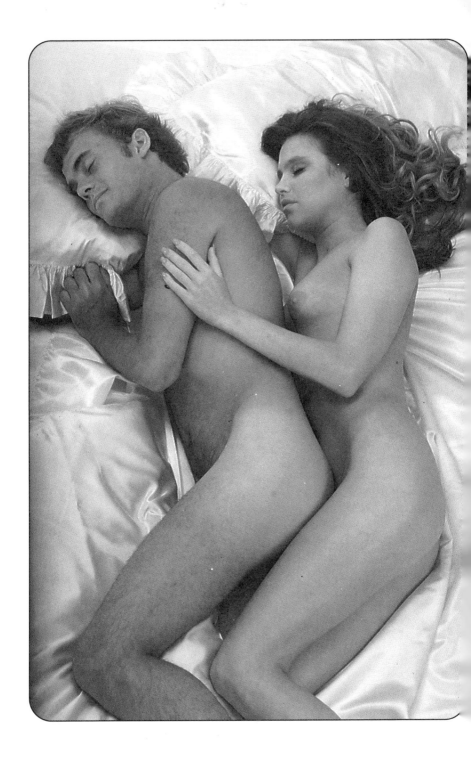

THE COUPLE AND CONTRACEPTION

Today's methods: some practical advice for making the best choice

NATURAL METHODS AND CONTRACEPTIVE PRODUCTS

To be able to choose the moment when one wants a child is a couple's absolute right and a decision which must be taken together and with mutual agreement. If this fundamental liberty is nowadays available to everyone, this is due to the scientific progress applied in the field of methods of contraception.

Contraception allows men and women to enjoy their sex life without feeling threatened by an unwanted pregnancy and knowing that contraceptive methods are not irreversible and that one only has to suspend their use to regain fertility.

THE PILL AND PILLS

This is what one also calls oral contraception: taking by mouth pills generally containing a mixture of hormones, oestrogens and progesterone, synthetic products but ones that are very close to natural female hormones.

The pill blocks ovulation, prevents the formation of the mucus that enables the spermatazoons to penetrate the uterine cavity and thins the uterine mucous membrane which is no longer able to form the 'nest' for an egg. Thus pregnancy becomes impossible.

There are different types of pills:

* **Sequential** – presented in strips of twenty-one (or twenty-two) pills, the first fourteen containing solely oestrogens and the last seven or eight a mixture of oestrogens and progesterone. These pills are only prescribed in special cases. They are 98 per cent effective.

* **Combined** – presented in strips of twenty-one pills, all containing a mixture of progesterone and oestrogens. They are 100 per cent effective.
* **Micro-pill** – presented in strips of twenty-eight pills containing only a very weak dose of progesterone. There can be a 1-2 per cent chance of failure.
* **Mini-pill** – containing a mixture of oestrogens and progesterone in minimal doses. They are 100 per cent effective.

Not every type of pill is suitable for every woman and the choice lies with the doctor. Any prescription only follows a complete examination. Questions will cover any history of cardio-vascular illness in the family, high blood pressure, diabetes and breast cancer. Tests will be taken for blood pressure and lung function. There is the smear test, as well as urine and blood tests to check cholesterol and sugar levels.

Formal contra-indications to the pill include pulmonary embolism (blood clots in the pulmonary veins), phlebitis (inflammation of the veins in the legs and the forming of a blood clot), a high cholesterol or glycaemia (blood sugar) level and breast cancer.

Any woman who is taking the pill must let her doctor know if she has any trouble with her periods. These could involve any bleeding, migraines, feelings of dullness and increases in weight of more than two kilos. A change in the hormonal dose or the prescription of a different make of pill will quickly sort out the problems.

Where she forgets to take a pill, the woman will have to take this pill as soon as she remembers.

THE COIL

This little device is placed by the doctor inside the uterus. There are several models in various sizes and shapes. Nowadays plastic coils are no longer used, except those with a leather thread. Some carry a reservoir containing progesterone. The possible failure rate of the coil has been put at 0.3-1.3 per cent.

Contra-indications include an infection of the uterus, vagina or Fallopian tubes, cancer of the genital organs, the start of pregnancy, bleeding outside the time of periods, congenital malformation of the uterus and certain fibroids.

The gynaecological examination enables the doctor to determine whether the coil is, in each particular case, suitable as a means of contraception. And it is he who puts this little apparatus, measuring about three centimetres, in place. This takes around five minutes and causes for a few seconds a light pain comparable to that felt at the start of a period.

A test-thread, very thin and supple, protrudes from the opening of the neck of the uterus. This enables the woman to check the presence of the coil and for the doctor to withdraw it at the end of its usable life – about four years for a standard model and eighteen months for one with a progesterone reservoir. It can equally be withdrawn should it prove unsuitable and, of course, if the woman decides she wants to become pregnant.

A medical check is necessary from two to four weeks after the coil's insertion and again every six months.

The presence of a well-positioned coil does nothing to impede sexual intercourse and equally does not prevent the use of a tampax.

When this apparatus is first used, periods will often be longer and more abundant, with the risk of small amounts of bleeding. But such inconveniences will disappear at the end of four or five months.

How the coil works can be summarised as follows: the presence of a foreign body modifies the composition of the mucus, which becomes incapable of guaranteeing the passage of spermatozoons and changes the uterine mucous membrane by reducing its capacities for providing a nest for any eggs.

THE DIAPHRAGM

This is a kind of cap in rubber or plastic whose edge, which is thicker, contains supple mini-springs to make its positioning easier. The cap covers over the neck of the uterus and provides a barrier against the spermatozoons, thus making fertilization impossible.

A gynaecological examination enables the doctor to determine the exact dimensions of the diaphragm. During the consultation the woman will be taught how to put it in place herself, after it has been coated with a spermicidal cream.

The diaphragm must be inserted up to two hours before sexual intercourse and should be left in place for between six and eight hours afterwards. In the event of repeated love-making, the diaphragm should be coated with spermicidal cream each time.

The doctor will recommend that the diaphragm is not left inside for more than twenty-four hours and this practical advice should be followed in order to keep it in good condition. Its useful life is about two years and its efficiency about 98 per cent, provided that it is used correctly.

This method is certainly quite exacting, since it requires a lot of practice to insert the diaphragm properly. But it does offer the advantage – and an important one for a lot of women and couples – of being natural, of not interfering with the physiological mechanism of the cycle.

There are a few contra-indications: a prolapse of organs, allergies to rubber or plastic and infections of the vagina or the neck of the uterus.

SPERMICIDES

In the form of creams, gels, foams, pessaries, pastes and soluble films, these are chemical products that literally 'kill' the spermatozoons that ejaculation deposits in the bottom of the vagina. Such a method of contraception is 95 per cent efficient and completely innocuous.

It is very rare to find cases of allergies with these products. They are applied locally before being put at the bottom of the vagina between ten and twenty minutes before intercourse.

This time, the method of application and the length of protection do vary according to the type of product chosen.

Gels, creams and pastes, which come in tubes with a vaginal applicator, should be used two or three minutes before the sexual act and will remain effective for between twenty minutes and one hour.

Pessaries should be introduced, by hand, about ten minutes before intercourse and their protection lasts between twenty minutes and one hour.

Foams, which are sold in aerosol cans fitted with an applicator, can be used at the time, without any waiting period. They keep their effectiveness for anything from half-an-hour to one hour.

As for soluble films, they are also applied by hand less than thirty minutes before having sex and protect for the same amount of time afterwards as the foams.

THE CONDOM

If the methods we have so far mentioned make the woman uniquely responsible for her contraception, then the condom puts this under the responsibility of the man.

The method is simple: the sperm held in the condom does not penetrate into the female's genital organs. And it is 100 per cent efficient if the instructions on its use are respected.

These involve unrolling it along the erect penis before penetration; gentle manipulation to avoid any risk of tearing it, however minimal this might be; immediate withdrawal after ejaculation; and only using the same condom once.

There is a vast range of makes on the market, which has grown considerably since the arrival and spread of AIDS. The choice must be of a brand sold in a chemist, carrying the 'kite' mark which certifies it has been tested to a minimum standard for strength and imperviousness.

The final date for use indicated on the wrapping is not obligatory, but it is interesting to know it, as it is the dimensions and the thickness of the rubber.

And some are lubricated and others even scented. So the couple will be able to try different ones before deciding which suits them best and is the most comfortable without diminishing any erotic sensations.

THE TEMPERATURE METHOD

During the period of ovulation, the couple must abstain from any sexual intercourse. And to ensure that she is aware of exactly when this occurs, the woman needs to check her temperature.

In effect, the ovaries secrete oestrogen hormones from the start of the period up to the day of ovulation, that is to say from the first to the fourteenth day of the cycle. From this moment and right up to the end of the cycle, the secretion of progesterone is added to that of oestrogens.

Progesterone has the peculiarity of raising the morning temperature by some tenths of a degree, which enables one to 'target' with precision the moment of ovulation.

To be effective (statistics indicate about 9 per cent failure), the method must be carried out very rigorously: taking one's temperature each morning at a fixed time, before getting up and in a lying-down position, and writing the result on a piece of graph paper.

The temperature is generally less than 37°C from the first day of the period to ovulation and equal to or more than 37°C from ovulation to the first day of the next period.

The period of infertility is between the eighteenth and twenty-eighth day of the cycle. Thus any safe intercourse is limited to about ten days.

While this method is certainly inconvenient, it does have the advantage of being completely natural.

WITHDRAWAL OR COITUS INTERRUPTUS

As with the condom, this method of contraception is placed under the responsibility of the man. For it is he who must withdraw quickly from his partner's vagina at the moment when he is about to ejaculate. As a result, the spermatozoons will not be in contact with the mucus of the neck of the uterus, thus avoiding the risk of fertilization.

Again, the man must have perfect control over his ejaculation, which is not always the case. Moreover, during intercourse, some secretion can escape from the meatus of the penis before the actual ejaculation. And the danger here is that this secretion often contains spermatozoons, which are fertilizing.

And finally, the practice of coitus interruptus means that intercourse cannot be repeated because, after the first contact, some spermatozoons may rest in the urethra and could then enter the vagina.

This explains the failure rate of this method, which statistically is as high as 30 per cent.

Moreover, from a sex point of view, it is quite inconvenient. There is the obligation on the part of the man to control himself while he reaches the point where he feels real pleasure. And there is the anxiety that this can provoke which often leads to a sense of frustration. As we have already seen, this means of contraception can be a cause of premature ejaculation.

For her part, the woman can equally feel worried, with the fear that her partner might not withdraw in time. And to this concern about the risk of an unwanted pregnancy one can add the absence of erotic sensations which, in some cases, spurts of sperm entering the vagina can cause.

SOME TESTIMONIES

Alice (age 27)

"We had discussed long and hard before our marriage and had decided to wait at least three or four years before having our first child. This would give us time to establish our financial situation and thus be able to pay for somewhere to live where the baby could have its own room and we could also enjoy some comfort.

"After a rigorous examination, my gynaecologist put me on the pill for a three-month trial. I had twenty-one pills to take for twenty-one days, then stopping for seven days so I would have my period. I told him that these were less abundant than before. I reminded him of this when I went back after the three-month trial. He reassured me, explaining that it was because of the hormonal content of the pill. So I continued to take them, without any inconvenience, and also to revisit my gynaecologist every six months.

"Then the moment came when Vince and I felt very strongly not only the desire to be parents but also the need to have 'our' child. That was three years after our marriage. Vince had been promoted at work. So had I. So I simply stopped taking the pill and, three months later, I was pregnant."

Maureen (age 26)

"Our little Nadine was born nine months – almost to the day! –after we made love for the first time. A real love-child, but the delivery was difficult. They had to cut round the vulva so that she could pass through. That was followed by a long period of extreme fatigue and even depression.

"I was just twenty and the idea of suffering again like that put me off the thought of getting pregnant again. I considered asking the doctor to put me on the pill. When I spoke to Ivan, he was horrified. He would never let me 'cheat' nature. He told me that women were made to have children and that the pill would make me ill – even bring on cancer! In short, he was totally opposed to the idea.

"I stood my ground and went to see a gynaecologist. From him I learned that the pill was not suitable for all women, that it involved a preliminary examination and that, if it could be prescribed, it sometimes brought on temporary troubles such as small amounts of bleeding between periods and headaches. I also found out recent studies had shown that, taken continually and with a high dose of oestrogens, there was a risk of developing cancer of the breast or uterus.

"This risk does not exist in today's pill, with lower doses, and the addition of the other female sexual hormone, progesterone. Besides, regular medical checks which people taking the pill must have allows for systematic detection of cancer.

"All this made me reflect hard and gave me the courage to bring the subject up again with my husband. He loves me and I love him. He understood that, like him, I wanted to have other children – but only when I was mentally and physically ready. I succeeded in convincing Ivan to come with me to the gynaecologist, who gave him all the assurances necessary for him to accept that I took the celebrated pill. That was two years ago. Now I want, we want another baby . . . So I am giving up the pill."

Matilda (age 33)

"I was on the pill for some years. No problem, except that more and more often I was forgetting to take it . . . In fact, I'd had enough of this programmed constraint. So, after a long session with my doctor and with his agreement, I chose to change my method of contraception and wear a coil. We made the appointment to have it fitted.

"When the day came, I was in an indescribable state of anxiety. First the doctor gave me a thorough examination. Then, while

I was still on the table with my legs apart, he slid a speculum (a special surgical mirror) into my vagina and placed a clip on the neck of the uterus. He explained fully as he went along what he was doing. I felt a little pain, but this lasted barely a few seconds.

"Then he took the coil out of its box and showed it to me – a small, very supple device in the shape of a 'V'. He put it into a thin plastic pipe fitted with an applicator. The coil was folded up to get it into the pipe, which the doctor then pushed into my stomach as he worked the applicator. At the same time he explained to me that, once free of the pipe, the coil would regain its initial shape and position itself in the uterus. I felt a little pain in the stomach.

"All that lasted about five minutes, although to me it had seemed interminable. The doctor then took out the clip and the speculum. It was over. I began to relax. He finally showed me the piece of thread that came out of my vagina and explained its purpose. I felt a little odd at the thought of having a foreign body inside me. However, the coil didn't bother me. It was just the idea in my head, which happily disappeared quite quickly. Now my coil and I are good companions."

Angela (age 39)

"My husband is an officer in the merchant navy, which means long periods of absence. Fortunately we have four children who really fill my life. After the fourth was born, we decided the family was complete. So, contraception for me.

"Neither the pill nor the coil struck me as particularly suited to a woman who spent several weeks and sometimes more without having intercourse. The withdrawal method we practised on occasions left me with frustrating memories. On the advice of my gynaecologist, I decided on the diaphragm, naturally after having been examined to make sure that there were no contra-indications.

"Now my diaphragm and the indispensable spermicide are at my disposal in the bathroom next to our bedroom and I have learned to place it as my doctor showed me, standing up with one knee bent and the foot resting on a stool. To begin with, I had a few difficulties. So I made the most of one of my husband's trips to get used to the technique. Now, in a few seconds, I discreetly put it in place before rejoining my husband who, each time he comes home, wants to make love to me as if we were twenty-year-olds."

Cynthia (age 31)

"Before taking the pill, which I have now been doing for seven years, I used to use spermicides. Like me, Simon found this a simple and practical method. We use to make love in the evening before going to sleep. I used a product which I had to put deep in my vagina three or four minutes before having intercourse. To do that, I had to lie stretched out on my back. During these minutes of waiting, Simon caressed my breasts, my stomach . . .

"And then one day I found I was pregnant. The doctor told me I must have used the spermicide incorrectly. But I had done it the same as always . . . Except that I then remembered one exception where we had made love in the morning. As I had to get to work, I proceeded to wash my vagina without waiting the eight hours prescribed in the method of use for the product, which therefore had not had time to fulfil its role of destroying the spermatozoons. And that was why, nine months later, we were the happy parents of little Jonathan!"

Pamela (age 29)

"We have been married for six years and have two children, both of whom Edward and I wanted. After each of my pregnancies – and even now – we have practised coitus interruptus as our method of contraception. I find it is better than putting some chemical product into my body or objects such as a coil or diaphragm, which I consider upsetting.

"But there is a small point which grieves me and that's Edward's need to pull himself free of me just at the moment when I really want him to push his penis even deeper inside me, even if I have already had an orgasm. I feel a sort of wrench, an insufficiency . . ."

Celia (age 32)

"Colin and I are practising catholics. If we have chosen the temperature method to limit the size of our family, it is because it is accepted by the Church. Certainly it is somewhat demanding to have to take my temperature every morning and especially to have to do it before getting up to see if our children are still asleep or even before going to get a glass of water! But, in the end, it is a habit that has become part of my daily life.

"There is one potential problem, however, which I experienced when a sore throat brought on a slight fever. I thought ovulation had started, when in fact it had not yet occurred. I found myself pregnant. But as this happened at the time when Colin and I had decided to try for a third child, the incident was of course welcome. Now, however, when I catch a cold or get toothache, I trust neither my thermometer nor my temperature chart. We wait until the last two days of the cycle before having sex. Happily such events rarely occur because, even if sensual caressing occupies an important place in our sex life, Colin and I have a strong need to make love."

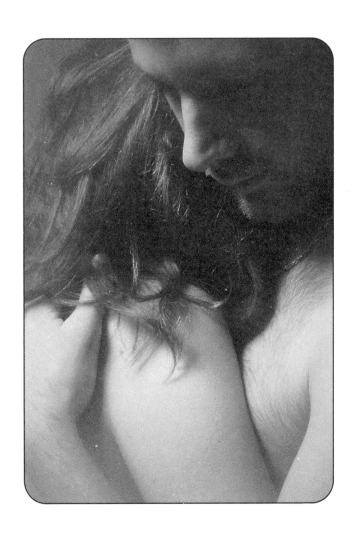

LIFE AND LOVE AFTER FIFTY

How to look after one's body and sexual health in order to remain young despite the passing years.

ARRIVING AT MIDDLE AGE

For women, to be on the wrong side of fifty means the time of menopause. Testimonies on this subject vary. For some the end of periods is a relief. For others it represents the loss of femininity, the knell of one's sex life.

According to the enquiry *Fifty Years, Long Live Life* carried out by Dr David Elia, for 60 per cent of woman the end of periods is seen as the end of a constraint, a real plus. They feel they have gained their freedom. On the other hand, the same enquiry showed that for 22 per cent it represents the loss of their youth.

SOME TESTIMONIES

Martine (age 51)
"From the age of twelve, each month I felt ill, with chest pains and a fatigue that wore me down for four or five days, the length of my periods. Now that they've finished, I can breathe a sigh of relief. Granted I can no longer have a child. But that for me is no problem, since I have two daughters and a son."

Laura (age 50)
"Menopause has given me a real sense of freedom. I no longer have the pressure of those periods which, without being really difficult, changed my humour and upset me. What's more, I am not tied to contraceptives anymore. I find both these points very positive."

Lucy (age 53)
"Good riddance! My husband has always been a fiery lover. And

having to stop having sex for almost a week every month used to make him even more impatient to make love, something that had cemented our relationship as a couple through twenty-seven years of married life. Now we are free to do it all the time."

Christine (age 55)

"When my periods started to become irregular and then stopped completely, I felt at a loss, melancholic, as if something had snapped inside me. I was entering another stage of my life, that of old age. I had to struggle against it, to rediscover the necessary energy to prevent letting myself go, to busy myself and make the effort to be always well-groomed, made-up and dressed. I finally got over being the wrong side of fifty after having touched on depression. Now I feel fine inside."

Paula (age 50)

Paula went through a similar experience. Her periods stopped early – between forty-seven and forty-eight. She did not even dare tell her husband for fear of appearing to him an old woman. She went as far as simulating each month the start of her period, wearing the necessary items and complaining of having swollen and painful breasts.

Finally, after two years, since menopause had not altered either her dynamism or her physical appearance, she abandoned this ridiculous charade and quietly accepted her physiological transformation.

WHAT HAPPENS AT MENOPAUSE?

It is important to understand the phase of premenopause – or perimenopause – which precedes menopause proper.

For 25 per cent of women premenopause comes between the ages of forty-two and fifty. It reveals itself in irregular periods, shorter cycles, lasting from twenty to twenty-five days instead of the usual twenty-eight, profuse periods, an increase in appetite leading to an increase in weight and swelling and pain in the breasts.

So what causes these different problems?

The ovaries, which have been functioning since puberty, suffer from fatigue and this effects the production of hormones. The ovaries produce too many oestrogens and not enough progesterone. It is this hormonal imbalance which upsets women during premenopause.

Meanwhile, the ovaries continue to lay eggs. So for those who want to avoid pregnancy, some method of contraception is still necessary.

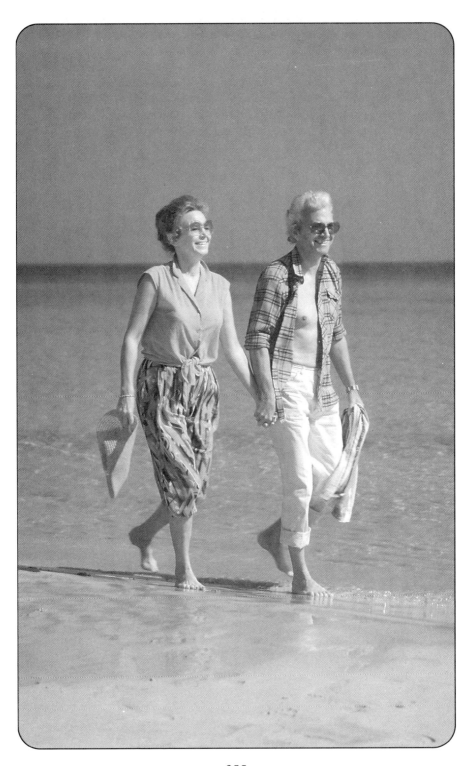

Can one counteract the disagreeable aspects of pre-menopause, which do have repercussions, however minor they may be, on one's sex life? The answer is to consult a gynaecologist, who will recommend a completely effective treatment to restore the equilibrium.

Menopause comes between forty-five and fifty-five – early at forty-five and late at fifty-five. Its medical definition is the complete stopping of periods for a year. The ovaries no longer produce either hormones or eggs.

Over-heating, heavy perspiration, insomnia, fatigue, drying of the vagina, reduction or loss of sexual appetite and sometimes painful intercourse – all these are among the symptoms that accompany the psychological upheaval.

While many generations of women have learned to accept menopause, today we know how to treat it through hormonal therapeutics and also mild medicines. There again, it is necessary to consult a gynaecologist who will adapt the treatment to the individual patient.

The majority of women who have undergone such treatment are able to rediscover their youth and afterwards live their sexuality without fear of an unwanted pregnancy.

MEN AS WELL . . .

"I am fifty-five and have been married twenty-eight years to a woman six years my junior. We are a happy couple, without hang-ups and with a good understanding about everyday things of life, such as work, leisure and sexuality. We make love frequently, about twice a week, which I believe isn't bad at our age.

"But for some time now I have felt a sort of lethargy, a lack of tonus, even over the question of sex. The pattern of our love-making is slowing down – I have to say because of me – and that is upsetting my wife."

This letter from Philip reflects the preoccupations of a great number of men of his age.

The fifties and sixties represent a stage in life that is sometimes difficult for a man to get through, too. It has often been compared to menopause in women and is described as andropause.

We should make it clear that some men cope with being the wrong side of fifty without any difficulty. Others complain of a loss of sexual appetite, problems with erection and very little resistance to fatigue. However, the male sexual organs continue to function normally (save in the case of particular illnesses) up to a very advanced age and even till the end of one's life.

Thus spermatozoons are produced permanently. Of course, their fertilizing power diminishes. But it has been known for men to become fathers in their late seventies and even after that. The testicles do not stop producing the male hormone testosterone. Thus no biological event can upset the sex life of men as they reach old age.

So where do the problems and difficulties that some complain of come from?

One can only lay the blame on the general ageing of the body which manifests itself in the putting-on of weight, slow digestion, lighter sleep and even insomnia, loss of memory and a slowing-down of reactions and mental capabilities. All this weighs on the mind of the individual who finds it hard to accept the progressive deterioration of his sexual capacity.

Generally one will point to the lethargy that sets in with a couple living together for a number of years who have not known how to introduce into their love-making the variety that is indispensable for the long life of their mutual enjoyment.

It is thus necessary to reawaken love, to indulge in manual or oral caressing and above all not to give up the practice of the sexual functions. "Men only become impotent when they abandon or neglect their genital faculties", wrote the Austrian psychiatrist Wilhelm Steckel, a disciple of Freud.

There are specific treatments to counteract the lowering of the sexual appetite. And as far as this is concerned there is no question of self-medication. It is imperative that one consults a specialist.

The taking of hormone-based medicines can prove effective. They relieve the state of depression and improve the sexual functioning. But hormonal therapy is not successful in every case and it is possible that some patients will register absolutely no positive results.

On the other hand some simple treatments, based on stimulants, vitamins or mineral salts are often sufficient to give energy and optimism to those men who are worried about their virility. They can rediscover, in a renewed zest for life, the taste for a new sexuality, rich in fantasies, imaginative games and sexual refinements.

LOVE AFTER FIFTY

There is no age at which one stops loving!

There are plenty of examples of couples who continue to enjoy a regular sex life well after seventy. If age reduces, for the woman as for the man, the sexual function – the same, moreover, as the other vital functions of the body – sexual activity is one of those that best resists the advancing of years.

REACTIONS OF THE MALE SEXUAL ORGANS

During the phase of excitement, it takes a man of over fifty two or three times longer to gain a full erection. It is necessary to count on about fifteen seconds, which is still an extremely short period of time. But it will get proportionately longer as one gets older. Among those over sixty it is possible to notice, during the plateau stage, a decrease in the length and size of the penis just before ejaculation, which is itself weaker and has less force.

This, however, does not alter the sexual pleasure. The contractions that set off the release of sperm still occur every 0.8 seconds, but the number is reduced to just one or two. Here we should remember that with young men sperm is released in three or four powerful spurts, followed by less forceful emissions of sperm which can last for several seconds.

Men of a certain age do benefit from being able to keep their erection longer before ejaculating. They have, moreover, a better control over their ejaculation than those who have not yet reached their fifties.

We should make two very positive points here, because they enable on the one hand the extension of foreplay and on the other that of coitus.

After making love, men over sixty experience an immediate – or almost immediate – deflation of the penis. A second erection is rarely possible for several hours. Quite clearly, however, sexual reactions will vary from one individual to another and depend on one's state of health.

One must stress that to maintain the sexual drive and the capacity to realise it, men must have regular sexual activity. As far as this is concerned, they must never 'take retirement'. Under such circumstances, one can understand the importance of the partner's behaviour, too.

HOW WOMEN CHANGE

Women over fifty have normally gone through menopause. We have already spoken about the psychological repercussions of the ending of periods, which give them the feeling that they have lost their femininity and that their sex life is over.

In fact, after their fifties, woman find themselves freed from most of the worries they previously experienced – notably their children's education and professional problems. In some way they feel more liberated in themselves. A lot then go through a rejuvenation of sexual desire. Those who have the courage to make their partner understand this will draw the most benefits.

So what happens to the female sexual organs after menopause?

The clitoris remains erectile and very sensitive to caressing. The vagina stretches more slowly during intercourse, its diameter reduces and the congestion of the external third becomes less intense. At the moment of orgasm, contractions occur from three to five times (five to ten times with a young woman).

After menopause, women often suffer a lack of lubrication and a reduction of the vaginal walls which can make intercourse painful. This problem is solved by hormonal treatment of which one can never say enough concerning the benefit it can have on women's sexuality and psyche.

THE DIFFICULT AGE

To be sure, with a couple who have had twenty-five or even more years of life together, love-making becomes less frequent. The reasons for this include a drop in libido, the tendency to tire more easily and problems of health which can arise with ageing.

However, there are those couples well into their sixties and beyond who continue to have very satisfying sexual intercourse because throughout the years they have known how to avoid the sexual lethargy and have kept up 'the flame of desire' by introducing a stimulating variation into their relationship.

It is with these couples that the difficult age has the least effect, this irresistible inclination that suddenly tempts men and women of a mature age to look for younger partners with whom they can rediscover the youth they thought was lost.

If the difficult age only lasts a short time, there is still nevertheless a serious risk that the couple could be destablised. With the dawning of old age, the prospect of solitude is a real drama as sixty-three-year-old Audrey explains:

"Certainly, Edgar and I made love more often when we were in our thirties. And certainly I neglected to stir up his passion and as a result I feel guilty.

"He was sixty-four and due to retire the following year. He was still working in a large store where he was a department head. I soon learned from a 'kind soul' that he was very friendly with a sales woman of thirty-eight who had recently got divorced. I shut my eyes to this, believing that it couldn't last.

"But it did! Two years, during which time I strove hard to win him back, dressing very smartly, making advances . . . But all in vain. Edgar hadn't left me, but his absences became more and more frequent.

"Then I noticed that he had changed a lot. He was thinner, much quieter and seemed to have lost interest in everything. So I decided to speak to him. He cried as he told me that his friend had left him. What could I do, except listen and try to console and comfort him? For several months I was at the same time his mother, his daughter, his best friend and his sister.

"Edgar became a lot closer to me to the point that he would never leave me alone. At night, in bed, we slept locked in each others arms. And, at last, the sexual urge returned. Now, three years after the trouble started, we have a lot of pleasure together."

If the difficult age most often affects men, women are not insensible to it. It is often more difficult for them to accept old age, to examine their wrinkles in the mirror, to count their white hairs.

For those women who do not want to accept their age, the compliments, admiration and soliciting of a young man provides a really youthful tonic. This type of liaison, however, is rarely gratifying and the relationship quickly falls apart, often leaving those who felt time was going to stand still more distressed than before.

In our opinion love, when one has reached the wrong side of sixty, can only be lived in calmness. The time has gone for disturbances, jealousy, aggression. Couples must protect each other and be, for example, a little selfish over the family invasions and the demands of grandchildren.

To look after one's health becomes an absolute necessity, with one's sexual health depending on a general state of well-being. One should have regular medical check-ups. The practice of certain physical activities (such as walking or swimming) and water therapy are the best guarantees for keeping in shape.

As part of one's overall programme, it is important to avoid over-eating or too much alcohol. And for one's sexual energy, why not indulge in some natural stimulants such as plants, nutrients, vitamins and minerals.

PLANTS TO REAWAKEN THE SENSES

The use of such plants goes back as far as antiquity and in current times, where ecology is very much to the fore, there is a real revival of interest in them. Their tonic-giving properties react on all parts of the body and can stimulate the sexual appetite.

Angelica, the dried root of which is sold in powder form and can be found in herbalist shops, is used in this way. You prepare it as an infusion (5 ml/1 tsp for a mug of boiling water) and drink it twice a day.

You can also make an infusion with **cinnamon** (5ml/1 tsp to

500 ml/17 fl oz/2¼ cups of water), the quantity corresponding to the daily ration necessary to reactivate the force of love.

With crushed **juniper berries** (4 ml/1 tsp to 500 ml/17 fl oz/2¼ cups of water), you will obtain the same results.

Coriander seeds, which give an agreeable flavour to cooking, serve as a base for an uplifting and aphrodisiac alcoholic drink: 25 g/1 oz/¼ cup of coriander seeds put to soak in 1 l/1¾ pts/4¼ cups of *eau-de-vie* (or other 'natural' alcohol such as vodka), to which one adds after a month a syrup prepared with 225 g/8 oz/1 cup of cane sugar and two glasses of water. This liqueur must then be left a further three months before being drunk . . . in moderation! A small glass once a day will be enough to produce the desired stimulating effect.

To reawaken the sexual energy, try an infusion of **fennel** or **rosemary** (5 ml/1 tsp of fennel seeds or rosemary leaves in a mug of water).

Everyone knows that **mint** is a stimulant. But it only becomes really exciting when mixed in equal proportions with **cinnamon**: 50 g/2 oz/½ cup of fresh mint leaves, 50 g/2 oz/½ cup of cinnamon and 1 l/1¾ pts/4¼ cups of water, boiled for ten minutes then left to settle for a further ten minutes before being filtered. Limit yourself to one cup a day of this concoction, drinking it hot or cold.

Nutmeg can help erection. Add three pinches of nutmeg to some hot red wine flavoured with orange peel.

The reputation of **pepper** is well-known. On condition that the stomach can take it, you can use it ground or milled on your food, notably meat. **Chillies**, which have a burning taste, contain the same properties . . . and present the same gastric problems.

Ginger, with its peppery flavour, is a well-known sexual stimulant, whether fresh, dried or ground. You can use it sprinkled over marinated fish, mixed with yoghurt or fruit salad.

The modest **clove** can also excite your cooking. Stick some cloves into a lemon and leave this to soak in 1 l/1¾ pts/4¼ cups of red wine – a very effective appetiser for your love-making exploits.

Oats contain a substance that acts on the human sexuality as it does on horses! In the form of flakes, oats provide an excellent dynamic breakfast.

The aphrodisiac virtues of **celery** are renowned. Whether as in the common stick form or as celeriac, the most effective recipe is a consommé, using the green leaves. Boil these for 30 minutes in 1 l/1¾ pts/4¼ cups of salted water with five or six peppercorns.

Onion soup is also good for reawakening fading passions. Calcium, potassium, magnesium, copper, zinc and vitamins A, B, C and E give this modest vegetable its exciting power. Allow two hours' cooking for five or six large onions in 1 l/1¾ pts/4¼ cups of salted water.

Rich in mineral salts such as calcium, potassium and magnesium, **wheatgerm** also contains vitamin E which reacts favourably on the functioning of the sexual glands. Sold under different forms at the chemist, wheatgerm also forms a part of some diet preparations – for example biscuits, crispbreads and breakfast cereals.

To counteract fatigue and a lowering of the sexual appetite, there is a very active natural product – **pollen**, the male element of the flower, which carries notably phospohorus, potassium and vitamins B, C, D and E. You can take it as an infusion or mix it with food.

The wealth of vitamin B5 in **royal jelly** makes this an exceptional natural food which will combat ageing of one's organs and skin. The vitamin in effect intervenes in the metabolism and the production of sexual hormones. A treatment with royal jelly twice a year provides a real youthful tonic . . . on condition that it is used in its pure form – the most expensive and most difficult to find.

You can take vitamins of the group B – phosphorus, potassium and magnesium – in biological **yeast**, to which they give their invigorating properties. You can get this yeast from diet shops to sprinkle over raw or cooked vegetables or in capsule form from chemists.

MORE FOR THE SEXUAL TONIC

In order to defend itself against the ageing of all its organs, sexual ones included, the body needs vitamins, minerals and micro-elements which are provided by the food we eat but also from top-ups, which come in various forms and are available from chemists with or without a prescription, depending on individual cases.

The following are the most important in relation to our sexuality:

Vitamin E

Anti-ageing, comes in vegetable oils (notably wheatgerm oil), beans, fruit, vegetables, liver.

Vitamin A

Known especially for its role in the quality of night vision and in the make-up of bones and is necessary for the health of the sexual glands. Found in eggs, dairy products, all meats and seafood.

Selenium

A micro-element which destroys the free radicals responsible for ageing. Food provides selenium in the form of fish and 'whole' cereals. One can take it in the form of supplements prescribed by the doctor.

Copper

A mineral that helps in the conversion into energy of fats and carbohydrates. Its deficiency reduces one's energy and dynamism. Deficiencies can be compensated for with supplements prescribed by the doctor. One should eat foods rich in copper such as offal, seafood, peanuts and raw beans.

Phosphorus

A mineral that assures the nervous energy and considered by some as a light aphrodisiac, it plays an essential role in cell reproduction. Its deficiency leads notably to the loss of general and equally sexual health. Its principle food sources are meat, fish, seeds, peanuts and beans.

Iron

A metal that makes up the essential element of the haemoglobin, charged with carrying oxygen in the red blood cells. Its deficiency provokes chronic fatigue. With women, long and profuse periods create a loss of iron which must be compensated for by taking supplements prescribed by the doctor and by eating food rich in iron such as offal, fish, mussels and poultry.

Magnesium

A mineral indispensable for the fabrication of chromosomes – and thus life. Its deficiency brings on cramp, spasms, feelings of stress and also a loss of sexual appetite. One also sees difficulties with erection among men suffering from its deficiency. A balanced diet will give the body the necessary amount of magnesium for it to function properly. Food that contains the most magnesium includes raw vegetables, cereals, milk and seafood. One can also take magnesium in tablet, granular or other forms, sold in chemists.

RECIPES FOR ROMANTIC OCCASIONS

Here are some delightful food ideas with aphrodisiac qualities to savour in the intimate surroundings of a candlelit room.

Choose fresh ingredients and simple recipes: anything too complicated will distract your attention. Anything too spicy or too heavy will take away, not enhance, desire. Think light and imaginative in your choice, and make sure your selection of courses complement one another perfectly.

Think about the presentation of the food. Colour and texture are vital. Aroma, too, can be immensely evocative. Present the food so that it looks beautiful and is a pleasure to see. Prepare it so that it is easy to eat. No one wants to battle with fish bones or too many crunchy ingredients. Deal with all that before you come to the table. Add some dishes that are meant to be eaten with your fingers – that can be very sensuous. Provide small finger bowls of warm water with a slice or two of lemon, and plenty of strong napkins.

Atmosphere is crucial. Set an attractive table, add relaxing music and soft lighting. Above all, avoid rush and hurry. Relish the flavours in warm and relaxed surroundings that set the mood for the occasion.

Appetisers and accompaniments

Appetisers are meant to whet the appetite for what is to come – and remember that you are thinking about more than just the food. Keep it delicate and sensuous.

Serve lightly steamed asparagus dripping with butter.

Serve crevettes in a light butter sauce or, of course, fresh oysters.

Prepare delicate swirls of wafer-thin salmon with a touch of cream cheese and topped with caviar.

Offer individual salmon mousses with the thinnest of melba toasts.

Serve light accompaniments such as steamed vegetables with a touch of melting butter on top; or beautifully prepared salads.

Mousseline à la coriandre
Coriander potato mousse
Dry fry 15 ml/1 tbsp coriander seeds in a pan until golden, shaking all the time. Boil and mash potatoes with plenty of butter and cream, then whisk them until very smooth. Pipe, if you like, into tiny swirls and bake in a hot oven for about 10 minutes until crisp on the outside while melting inside.

Main courses
Forget the crispy roasts or dense casseroles. Remember lightness of touch. Meat should be so tender it almost dissolves in the mouth. Seafood often offers a light alternative.

Try salmon steaks, skinned and with the bones lifted out after cooking, with a wine sauce.

Cook a perfect steak – only if you can cook a perfect steak – to serve with an unctuous, very gently spiced sauce.

Cailles au genièvre
Quails with juniper
Lightly fry 2 quails in a little butter until golden. Sprinkle with 45 ml/3 tbsp gin and flambé by setting a match to the alcohol. Lightly crush and add 10 juniper berries and freshly ground salt and pepper. Cover and cook gently for about 10 minutes until the birds are cooked. While the quails are cooking, cut two large slices of bread, remove the crusts and fry the bread lightly in a little butter on both sides until golden brown. Arrange the bread on warm plates and sit the quails on top. Add 60 ml/4 tbsp of cream to the quail cooking juices and heat stirring, for 1–2 minutes. Pour over the quails and serve.

Magret pimentés
Spicy duck breasts
Remove the skin from the duck breasts and fry them in butter for about 20 minutes until cooked. While they are cooking, chop a chilli, an onion and a garlic clove and fry them in a little oil until browned. Soak 50 g/2 oz/½ cup breadcrumbs in a little milk and stock so that it creates a paste. Stir this into the onion mixture, season with salt and simmer for 15 minutes, adding a little more stock or water if the sauce is too thick. Pour over the duck to serve.

Fondue aux truffes
Truffle fondue
Put 225 g/8 oz grated cheese, 50 g/2 oz/¼ cup butter and some salt and pepper in the top of a double saucepan and heat over boiling water, stirring to a soft paste. Gradually add 2 egg yolks, then a thinly sliced truffle. Serve with cubes of bread lightly fried in butter to dip into the fondue sauce.

Huîtres chaudes au porto
Oysters in port
Remove 12 oysters from their shells and rinse well, then return them to their half-shells. Mix together 1 egg yolk, a glass of port, 60 ml/4 tbsp of fresh cream and season with salt and pepper and pour over the oysters. Bake in a hot oven at 200°C/400°F/Gas 6 for about 10 minutes.

Desserts
Forget anything heavy, anything too hot or too cold. Go for creamy desserts with a sensuous texture, served at room temperature or gently warm. A little alcohol in the mixture gives piquancy to the flavour. Another alternative is fresh exotic fruits, but have them ready prepared so they are easy to eat. Fresh figs or lychees, soft

peaches or nectarines, or a fruit salad prepared in bite-sized pieces in its own juice or a very light syrup.

Crème brulée à la muscade
Almond crème brulé
Bring 500 ml/17 fl oz/2¼ cups of milk to the boil with 25 g/1 oz/ 2 tbsp of sugar and a few pinches of freshly grated nutmeg. Beat 2 eggs in a bowl, then whisk in the hot milk and pour into a small flameproof baking dish. Stand the dish in a roasting tin half filled with boiling water and cook in the oven at 190°C/350°F/Gas 5 for about 30 minutes until the custard is just set. Sprinkle generously with ground almonds and brown sugar and brown under a hot grill until the sugar caramelises. Leave to cool.

Mousse au chocolat et aux épices
Chocolate brandy mousse
Melt 125 g/5 oz plain chocolate with 30 ml/2 tbsp brandy or whisky. Add a pinch of ground cloves, a twist of black pepper, 3 egg yolks, 125 g/5 oz/1⅔ cup melted butter and a dash of vanilla essence (extract) and mix well. Whisk 3 egg whites until stiff, then fold them gently into the mousse and chill. Serve not too cold with swirls of grated chocolate on the top.

Glace à la canelle
Cinnamon sorbet
Boil 600 ml/1 pint/2½ cups of milk with 5 ml/1 tsp ground cinnamon, then leave to cool. Whisk 5 egg yolks with 100 g/4 oz/ ½ cup caster sugar until the mixture turns pale and comes off the whisk in ribbons. Pour in the milk, stirring all the time. Heat the mixture gently, stirring until it thickens. Stir in 15 ml/1 tbsp vodka. Allow to cool. Pour into a freezer tray and freeze, stirring occasionally until solid. Transfer to the fridge an hour before serving in sorbet glasses with a sliver of lemon rind.

Crème médici
Sweet wine cream
Mix 3 egg yolks, a glass of white dessert wine, 50 g/2 oz/¼ cup caster sugar and about 2.5 ml/½ tsp ground cinnamon. Heat gently, whisking to a creamy consistency. Serve warm with *langue de chat* biscuits.

Drinks
Wines should complement the food you have chosen, but what better choice could there be than Champagne? If that is beyond your budget, there are many light sparkling wines with good flavour that you can try. Avoid anything too heavy or too sweet. Lightness of touch is everything.

9

MEDICAL FILE

•

Some brief but useful information about sexual physiology and health. In this chapter men, women and couples should find plenty of help and advice on how to understand and cope better with various medical issues that could from time to time affect them and thus gain a greater appreciation of the effects of certain everyday behaviour on their sexuality.

•

PROBLEMS FOR THE MALE

THE MALE SEXUAL HORMONES

These are produced from the age of puberty by the sexual glands. Called androgens, they are responsible for the physical changes that form part of adolescence: hair growth, breaking of the voice, broadening of the shoulders, development of the muscles . . .

At the same time the sexual urge is born and the first ejaculations commence. It is the testicles, these two egg-shaped glands hidden in the scrotum, that secrete these hormones, in particular the testosterone which is the principal male hormone. The testicles also assure the production of spermatozoons.

Unlike for a woman, where the sexual hormones respect a certain cycle, for a man the testosterone and the spermatozoons are produced on a permanent basis. With the passing of years, the rate of testosterone production decreases in proportions that do not normally affect one's sex life until an advanced age.

In the event that one does experience difficulties in this context, one should seek advice: the doctor will ask for a hormone check and look for the causes of this reduction. There can be two reasons: testicular insufficiency (which is very rare) or problems with the pituitary gland. One knows that it is this gland, found at the base of the brain, which through orders from the hypothalamus, the neighbouring nervous centre, sets off the fabrication of the testosterone. A suitable treatment will then be prescribed.

The whole medical profession is nowadays at one in acknowledging the dangers of testosterone injections. While this process is beneficial in the short term, prolonged treatment worsens the state of the patient and can lead to cancer of the prostate.

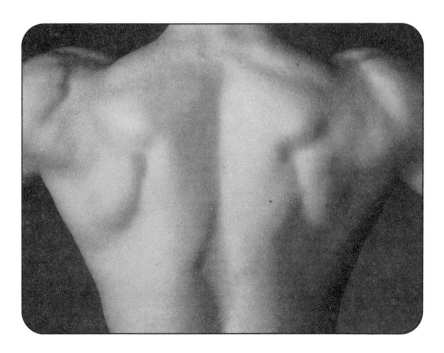

SPERM

This whitish sticky liquid, with a lightly chlorinated smell, is emitted from the penis at the moment of ejaculation. It is essentially made up of spermatozoons, produced by extremely thin tubes situated in the testicles. In fact they create about a million every day!

It is the spermatozoons which, during ejaculation, are projected to the bottom of the vagina where, thanks to the mucus from the neck of the uterus, they then penetrate inside and continue their progress towards the Fallopian tubes.

From the fourteenth day of the cycle, a certain number of eggs develop in the ovaries. Just one will reach maturity. It frees itself from its envelope, the follicle, and is absorbed by the enclosure of a Fallopian tube. A single spermatozoon is going to enter the egg and fertilize it. The two male and female elements will only constitute one element: the first cell of the future child.

Into the sperm's composition there also enters a creamy substance secreted by the seminal vesicles, two glands found above the prostate. Rich in fructose, it feeds the spermatozoons and enables them to move quickly.

To these secretions are added those of the two Cooper glands, found below the prostate, and the Littré glands, which are around the urethra. These provide the sperm with about a third of its composition in the form of a liquid called prostatic fluid.

Each ejaculation represents two to four cubic centimetres of sperm and each cubic centimetre contains anything from 50 to 200,000 million spermatozoons.

PHIMOSIS

This is a narrowing of the orifice of the foreskin, the thin membrane that covers the penis when resting and, under the effect of erection, allows it to pass through.

There are two types of phimosis – congenital and acquired. In the first case, phimosis is due to the fact that the foreskin is too tight, sometimes linked with a shrinking of the bride, the small ligament in the skin situated on the lower part of the penis. In the second case, phimosis results from an infection or adhesion between the penis and the foreskin.

Whatever its origin, phimosis makes masturbation and intercourse painful.

One can remedy this through a simple and safe operation: circumcision through surgery, which involves excising the foreskin. Thus the penis is permanently exposed. In certain parts of the world (some American states, Africa and Oceania), as with certain religions (Jewish and Muslim), circumcision is normally carried out at birth.

By removing the folds of the foreskin, one avoids the risks of infection brought on by insufficient hygiene and the presence of smegma, a whitish fatty secretion with an often disagreeable smell which accumulates under the foreskin.

In the case of the bride shrinking, which makes erection difficult and can even cause premature ejaculation, a small operation is needed. This consists of making a transverse incision of the ligament. Thus one eliminates the risk of laceration, something that is not in itself really serious but can lead to a rupture of the artery and a haemorrhage, which can cause concern.

When the penis is squeezed too tightly by the foreskin, the action involved in its release can provoke strangulation. This is known as paraphimosis, which is extremely painful and requires an urgent operation.

THE PROSTATE

This gland, which is to be found in the lower part of a man's stomach near the bladder, is crossed by the urethra. This duct, which runs the whole length of the penis, opens out at the end through a small orifice called the meatus through which flows the urine and sperm.

The prostate, the size and shape of a chestnut, makes the prostatic fluid that constitutes a third of the sperm's composition. It also has another sexual function: in the course of ejaculation, it contracts to propel the sperm into the urethra.

Its deep position makes a radiological examination difficult. To evaluate its volume and consistency in order to detect any eventual anomalies, the doctor will have to 'feel' it through the rectum. With his middle finger suitably 'dressed' and lubricated, he introduces it into the anus and feels the prostate through the wall of the rectum.

This examination is not painful and should be carried out systematically with all men over the age of forty-five. Through this one can discover if there is an adenoma, a benign tumour but one which, as it develops, causes trouble with urination, accompanied by the feeling of burning and pain in the lower abdomen. More serious, but relatively less common, cancer is also detectable.

Among the troubles one can have with one's prostate, we should mention inflammation, caused by the stagnation of sperm in the prostate which does not empty itself out totally during ejaculation, and infection through gonococcus. In about 85 per cent of cases, a specific medical treatment will be prescribed. If surgery is decided on and carried out under good conditions on a patient whose general state of health is satisfactory, there should be no dramatic repercussions.

Generally the sphincter of the bladder is suppressed and, during ejaculation, the sperm will be forced into the bladder. Thus there will be no external ejaculation and no chance of fertilizing one's partner. However, neither one's erection nor orgasm is reduced, nor the sensation of pleasure that accompanies the sexual act. A normal sex life can be restored after convalescence.

VASECTOMY

This is, in effect, male contraception through surgery and should only be carried out where it becomes absolutely necessary. A possible example would be the situation of a father of a large family whose wife cannot cope with any form of contraception and whose state of health no longer allows her to go through pregnancy and childbirth.

Any decision to have a vasectomy must only be taken after the most serious reflexion and with the advice of doctors and psychologists. The reason for this is that, while the operation is simple and without risk (it takes about a quarter of an hour under local anaesthetic), it is irreversible. The man will be sterile for the rest of his life.

However, vasectomy has no effect on the capacity for erection or orgasm or the pleasures it brings. Ejaculation will always occur, but the sperm does not contain any spermatozoons.

The operation consists of cutting the two ducts known as the deferent ducts, which carry the spermatozoons from the testicles where they are made as far as the prostate, where they are mixed with the fluid produced here to form sperm. An incision about a centimetre long is made in the skin of the testicles and the deferent ducts extracted to be sectioned or ligatured or submitted to electro-coagulation. They are then put back in place and the testicles resealed.

Generally the surgeon who operates suggests that the patient keeps his sperm in a special bank, just in case the situation should ever arise in the future whereby he might wish to 'fertilize' a partner. It would then be necessary to resort to artificial insemination.

SEXOLOGY AND GYNAECOLOGY

THE GYNAECOLOGICAL EXAMINATION

Plenty of women dread this, wrongly, because it is not painful. And it is absolutely necessary for checking on the condition of one's genital organs.

The woman lies on the examination table with her knees raised, her thighs apart and her feet supported in some stirrups. The doctor introduces a speculum into the vagina. This metal apparatus is made up of two 'tongues' closed together which can be opened with the use of a screw at the base.

The speculum is placed in the vagina in a closed position and then opened gradually. The doctor can thus examine the walls of the vagina and the neck of the uterus. He also takes a sample of the vaginal secretions and puts them on thin plates of glass. This is the vaginal smear. Analysis of this is carried out in a special laboratory.

The doctor then proceeds to 'feel' the vagina as far as the base, using two fingers covered with supple polythene. This enables him to assess the size, shape and direction of the uterus.

Since the normal length of the uterus is from four to six centimetres, anything more than this indicates pregnancy or a fibroma. With about 20 per cent of women, the uterus is tilted towards the back. This is known as retroversion, a peculiarity of the anatomy which is in no way serious and does not affect either one's sex life or reproduction.

At the same time the doctor checks the state of the ovaries. If they exceed their normal size – about three centimetres long and up to two centimetres wide – this can indicate the presence of a cyst.

Finally he checks that the Fallopian tubes are not accessible to the touch. One can only feel them in the event of an abnormal thickening due to infection.

This examination provides invaluable information and, where necessary, enables specific treatment to be carried out in each case.

ULTRA-SOUND EXAMINATION

This very commonly prescribed examination for checking on the state of the genital organs and pregnancy involves a technique using ultrasonic waves and not x-rays, as with radiography. Thus it carries no danger for either examiner or patient.

The high-frequency sound waves, which cannot be detected by the human ear, are absorbed during their passage through the organs, bones and tissues. By studying the beam of the ultrasonic waves reflected on the surface that separates two different media – for example, muscles and fluid – one can detect any possible anomalies in the organs.

Before undergoing this test, the patient will have to drink a litre and a half of water. This is to fill the bladder in order to push back the genital organs and to reflect the sound waves, which are captured and then form images on a small screen.

The whole process, which is absolutely painless, lasts between fifteen and thirty minutes, depending on individual cases, after which time the patient can immediately relieve her bladder.

By means of this scan one can measure the volume of fibromas and watch their growth. One can equally confirm the diagnosis of a cyst in the ovary and distinguish the type, whether organic or functional *(see pages 279-80)*.

Nowadays the whole period of pregnancy is monitored using this method. Thus the gynaecologist can follow the growth and vitality of the foetus, detect any possible anomalies, know the sex of the child and establish at an early stage whether there is to be a multiple birth.

LAPAROSCOPY

This recent method of exploring the abdominal cavity allows one to diagnose and eventually to conduct certain surgery without having to open up the wall of the abdomen.

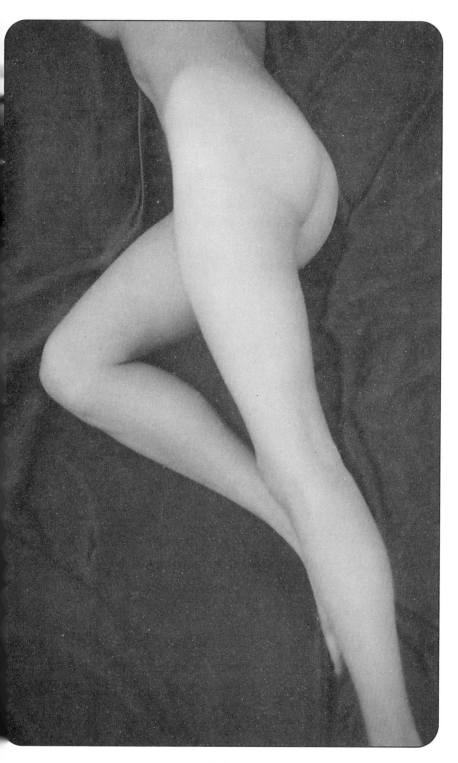

The technique is simple. Having anaesthetised the patient, the surgeon introduces a tube across the wall of the abdomen to blow in a gas designed to open the organs and thus see them better. The surgeon then makes a tiny hole at the level of the navel and introduces a rigid tube at the end of which is fitted a light and optical system. Thus he can see inside the stomach and examine the organs there.

With laparoscopy, it is possible to diagnose an ectopic pregnancy, a cyst in the ovary and other anomalies in the tubes and ovary often responsible for sterility.

Endometriosis is equally visible using laparoscopy. This complaint, characterised by the presence of small pieces of the uterine mucous membrane in other parts than the uterus (for example the tubes, ovaries or bladder), causes pain during periods and in the course of making love.

Once the diagnosis is made, the surgeon can operate if he feels it necessary. This can involve making a second 'buttonhole', in which he inserts flexible rods fitted with mini surgical instruments, or he introduces the instruments using the tube already in place.

The operation is carried out by the surgeon watching the optical system, where the image is projected on a video screen. We should underline the fact that, even though this is an operation, the patient will not be left with any scars.

Laparoscopy does require a short hospitalisation of three days. It is not a traumatising examination. After waking up and during the next forty-eight hours, the patient will feel some stiffness. And generally this is followed by a week's convalescence.

X-RAYING THE UTERUS

Hysterography, another examination that can be prescribed by the gynaecologist and one that involves the use of x-ray, is carried out to check the following:

* **the state of the uterus,** with the object of detecting a possible polypus, fibroma or even cancer.

* **the state of the Fallopian tubes,** with the object of finding the causes of sterility. Here one can see whether the tubes are clear or blocked or even dilated or thickened through the presence of an infection or an endometriosis.

The examination takes place during the week following a period. The patient lies on the table in the gynaecological position. The radiologist introduces into the duct passing the neck of the uterus a contrasting fluid that will facilitate the x-raying of the deep organs – the uterus and the Fallopian tubes. A vacuum is then created with the help of a nozzle or cupping-glass connected to a syringe filled with an iodized solution that is opaque to the X-rays. This solution is injected slowly into the uterus and passes into the tubes.

In principle this test should not be too painful. The woman will feel a slight stomach pain comparable to the one she has when her periods arrive. If the pain is severe, this indicates the presence of an infection.

Some women dread this test and arrive in an anxious or nervous state, which risks making it more painful. So it is necessary to be as relaxed as possible beforehand.

It can be that the gynaecologist prescribes a hysterography limited to the uterus, notably in the case of fibroma. The injected liquid is then restricted to the uterine cavity and does not pass into the Fallopian tubes. Thus any feelings of pain are largely reduced.

THE FEMALE SEXUAL HORMONES

These are secreted by the glands found in the internal and external genital apparatus. In the inner and outer lips the secretion from the Skène and Bartholin glands assures lubrication of the vagina, which is necessary for comfortable and successful intercourse.

Other glands placed in the vulva give it its specific smell, which a lot of men find very exciting.

It is the ovaries, two glands situated in the lower pelvis, which produce the two essential sexual hormones – oestrogens and progesterone.

These are produced from the age of puberty and are responsible for the physical, physiological and also emotional changes in a young girl: development of the breasts, curving of the hips, appearance of pubic hair, changes in the vulva, increase in the volume of the uterus, awareness of femininity and growing sexual and emotional urges.

Periods then follow and the young girl is capable of reproducing. From then on and right up to menopause, she will live under the influence of these hormones. During the fourteen days of the cycle, the ovaries are going to secrete exclusively oestrogens, then after the fourteenth day progesterone as well. The mucous membrane that lines the uterus will become impregnated and ready to receive the fertilized egg, if there has been an encounter between an ovule and a spermatozoon.

The oestrogens are equally responsible for the production, through the neck of the uterus, of the gluey mucus that assures the transport of the spermatozoons.

Again it is the sexual hormones that see pregnancy through to its culmination and also feed the sexual appetite.

Thanks to the most recent scientific discoveries concerning hormonal receptors on to which the specific corresponding hormones come to attach themselves, some new synthetic hormones have been put to the test. Thus, in the case of hormonal deficiency – at menopause, for example – synthetic hormones can substitute for the natural ones.

DRYING OF THE VAGINA

The lack of lubrication makes sexual intercourse difficult, provoking sores, irritations or itching which can create a fear of coitus. The partner also feels some unpleasant effects, the penetration of the penis often becoming painful.

Vaginal lubrication is normally provided through the sebaceous glands situated in the outer and inner lips, the sweat and Skène and Bartholin glands. Under the effects of sexual excitement, the walls of the vagina also emit a lubricating substance.

When this physiological phenomenon fails to occur, one must find out why. This means a visit to the gynaecologist.

Recurring genital infections, such as herpes, are often the origin of this problem, as can be a change in the circulation in the vaginal walls or even inflammation of the lubricating glands. Equally, the after-effects of a gynaecological operation may provoke drying of the vagina, as can those following a difficult childbirth necessitating the cutting of the vulva – known as episiotomy *(see page 278)*.

Deficiency of oestrogens (the female hormone) is also a source of drying of the vagina. This symptom very often occurs in the period of premenopause and menopause. The appropriate medical treatment generally brings good results. The use of a local lubricant is recommended in the majority of cases.

We should finally point out that excessive personal hygiene such as vaginal douches, the use of tampax and deep washing with disinfecting products all risk altering and drying the vaginal mucous membrane. Such a cause of the change in the lubricating process stops quickly once these habits are given up.

LACK OF PERIODS

Known by doctors under the name of amenorrhea, the lack of periods can be either primary or secondary.

Primary is where a woman has never had a period. The cause can be a genital malformation or the absence of an organ – the uterus, for example – or equally insufficient secretions from the hypophysis.

Genital anomalies are most often sorted out by surgery, although happily these are quite rare. Troubles with the hypophysis involve medical treatment, which has proved to be effective.

Secondary amenorrhea occurs with women who have previously had periods. It can quite simply be a question of pregnancy or early menopause. Psychological or emotional traumas (bereavement or divorce, for example) or exceptional fatigue can interrupt one's periods. However, these will be re-established through treatment of the causes, whether this involves psychotherapy or specific medicines.

Amenorrhea sometimes follows infectious illnesses (such as tuberculosis) which lead to a marked deterioration in one's general state of health.

Finally, endocrinal illnesses (such as diabetes) can also be responsible – for example, Basedow and Adison. There again, following diagnosis through a whole series of examinations, the doctor will decide what is the appropriate therapy.

Anyone who has gone three months without a period must consult a gynaecologist. The tests involved are not painful: taking one's temperature every morning, checking the prolactine level in the blood and taking doses of ovarian, suprarenal and hypophysis hormones. These will identify the causes of the problem and enable it to be treated, most often with success.

PAINFUL PERIODS

It is far from rare that both young and older women have painful periods from time to time. Gynaecologists call this dysmenorrhea. Some pain – small shooting pains and feelings of heaviness in the abdomen – is considered normal. But not when such pain is sharp and repeated each month. It is necessary to consult a gynaecologist to find out the causes of this problem.

In about 80 per cent of cases, the doctor will not detect any cause of pain. He will prescribe painkillers, which will have a soothing effect. These come in the form of capsules or tablets to take at certain times during the cycle, which he will identify.

In 20 per cent of cases, the doctor does discover the cause of dysmenorrhea. Its origin can be a gynaecological infection (a cyst in the ovary, for example) or endometriosis (*see page 280*). The diagnosis will be made on the basis of clinical tests or through an ultra-sound scan, hysterography or laparoscopy. A specific treatment will then be prescribed, the results of which are generally effective.

Another cause can be excessive secretion of prostaglandins, small molecules secreted by the mucous membrane that lines the uterus. This secretion provokes contractions of the uterus aimed at expelling the fragments of mucous membrane during periods. The excess secretion of prostaglandins intensifies these contractions which then become painful. A prescription of anti-inflammatories produces excellent results. These products suspend or slow down the secretion of prostaglandins.

A woman's suffering during each of her cycles brings on worry and tiredness which take their toll on both her humour and her relationship with her partner. Thus it is vital that one seeks immediate advice over such pains.

EPISIOTOMY

It can happen during childbirth, especially when the woman is having a baby for the first time and her vulva is less stretched than that of women who have already had one or several children, that the baby's head is too big to pass through without the vulva being torn. The 'natural' cut is in the form of 'saw-teeth' and the tear causes an unsightly swelling around the scar.

To avoid this inconvenience, the surgeon makes an incision several centimetres long from the vulva towards the anus. This is an episiotomy. Once the baby has been delivered, this opening is sewn up with special thread that dissolves after eight or ten days.

The woman is going to remain sensitive in this area and even suffer some pain, which will make her reluctant to have sexual intercourse or indeed refuse it. Such discomfort can last several weeks. If it continues, she must go and see her doctor who will decide whether the cut should be opened up again and redone. This surgery is not serious and normally only involves a few hours hospitalisation.

During the healing-up period, it will be necessary to clean the affected area daily with special products prescribed by the surgeon or doctor. And a regular medical check-up will ensure that any infection can be spotted and treated straight away.

FIBROMA

This is a benign tumour which develops on the wall of the uterus. It is a muscle composed of layers of muscular fibres about a centimetre thick. The uterus is hollowed out in a cavity and it is in this cavity that the foetus grows during pregnancy.

A gynaecological examination will reveal the presence of one or more fibromas, which can be the size of a ping-pong ball or grow to as much as twenty-five centimetres long.

We still do not know what causes a fibroma to form. Certain research tends to indicate that it corresponds to a hormonal imbalance. But one thing is agreed: fibromas most often occur in women whose mother has already had the problem and among women going through the stage of premenopause. Another extremely important point: a fibroma never grows into a cancer.

Indications of the existence of a fibroma include:

* long and heavy periods,
* bleeding outside periods and
* frequent desire to urinate (when the fibroma is large).

A fibroma can be responsible for sterility. Anyone who is suffering from abnormal bleeding must seek medical advice without delay. A regular check-up – on average twice a year – enables the doctor to keep an eye on the possible growth of fibromas. He may recommend an ultra-sound scan, which will show up precisely the size of any fibroma.

Where one or more exist, the size of which he considers 'reasonable', the gynaecologist will prescribe a hormonal medication to stop not only the growth of the fibroma but also the bleeding outside the time of periods. This treatment will have to be continued right up to menopause, the moment at which fibromas wither. Some even disappear completely.

Whether or not an operation is required will depend on the size of the fibroma and whether it continues to provoke bleeding outside periods. The operation involves either extracting the fibroma from the uterus (known as a myomectomy) or removing the uterus itself (known as a hysterectomy). Neither operation has any adverse effect on the sex life of the patient.

OVARIAN CYSTS

These are tumours that develop in the ovaries, two glands found in the lower abdomen either side of the uterus which produce the female sexual hormones – progesterone and oestrogens – and also the fertile ovule.

A distinction is drawn between the organic cyst and the functional cyst. The first, which contains organic waste (hair, teeth, blood, etc), risks deteriorating into a cancer. The second increases in size up to the time of a period then disappears for good or reappears up to the next period before disappearing again.

The cyst, which can reach the size of an egg and even that of a large orange, just contains fluid. Its presence, whether it is organic or functional, is sometimes indicated by bleeding and pains before a period and during sexual intercourse. It will normally be detected during a gynaecological test through palpation, the affected ovary forming a kind of swelling. An ultra-sound scan will confirm the presence of a cyst and enable one to tell whether it is organic or functional.

In the former case, it is necessary to operate. The removal of a cyst is carried out under general anaesthetic and involves opening up the wall of the abdomen (known as laparotomy). Sometimes the surgeon will have to remove the ovary at the same time. Such operations have no effect on the woman's sex life.

In the case of functional cysts, also called 'false cysts', medical treatment will generally be effective. This essentially consists of regularising the activity of the ovaries through the taking of pills or synthetic hormones.

ENDOMETRIOSIS

The uterus is a hollow muscle, the cavity of which is lined with a mucous membrane – the endometrium. This is the membrane that, impregnated throughout the cycle by oestrogens and from the fourteenth day up to the period itself by progesterone as well, forms the 'nest' in which the fertilized egg settles.

It is possible for fragments of this membrane to escape from the uterine cavity and find their way into other organs in the lower abdomen – for example the ovaries, the tubes, the uterus itself, the peritoneum or the intestine. This is endometriosis.

Normally, at the moment when the period starts, the uterine membrane bleeds and is released with the menstrual blood. In the case of endometriosis, the fragments of endometrium also bleed, causing pain in the organs on which they settle. And endometriosis also causes pains during intercourse and, in certain cases, provokes sterility.

Although a gynaecological examination with a speculum and a palpation check will enable the doctor to suggest a diagnosis, additional tests such as laparoscopy or hysterography *(see pages 272 and 274)* are often necessary.

The treatment can be medical: the prescription of high-dose hormones for several months, which will atrophy the centre of the endometriosis.

The recent discovery of a hormone secreted by the hypothalamus in the brain – the LHEV – has led to the application of a new hormonal treatment which stops the functioning of the ovaries completely. The result of this is also to atrophy the centre of the endometriosis.

In certain cases surgery will be necessary in order to remove the source of the problem which can otherwise form nodules on the genital or intestinal organs.

OSTEOPOROSIS

Following menopause, one woman in three is affected by osteoporosis – a decalcification of the bones and the vertebrae which can occur between five and ten years after the periods have stopped.

This causes back pains and bone fragility which in turn leads to fractures, notably the neck of the femur, which can occur after a fall or slight impact. Pains will then appear in the back and the lumbars. In some cases, a compression of the vertebrae can result, causing a reduction in size.

Osteoporosis develops in the following way:

With menopause, the ovaries stop functioning. The hormones – oestrogens and progesterone – are no longer secreted by the ovaries. The periods disappear and fertilization is no longer possible. The oestrogens, which help build up the bones, no longer play their role and can therefore not counteract the destructive action of the suprarenal hormones.

One can thus understand the essential role hormonal treatment plays here in compensating for the deficiency of oestrogens. There is an imbalance between the support and destruction of the bone structure, which is going to suffer from this imbalance – and from decalcification.

Osteoporosis and its effects can be prevented by following a diet rich in calcium (dairy produce and mineral waters full of calcium) or supplements of calcium in tablet form. Control over the amount of calcium in the bones is done by examination – bone densiometry. This is a special x-ray treatment using a scanner.

OVARIECTOMY

This is the removal by surgery of one or both ovaries, made necessary in certain cases such as cancer of the ovary, a very large cyst which has affected the whole of the ovary or the removal of the uterus following menopause.

Generally the surgeon tries, if the patient has not yet reached menopause, to save a fragment of the ovary tissue to avoid provoking a surgical menopause.

For it is the ovaries that secrete the female sexual hormones oestrogens and progesterone, which are responsible for the continuation of the cycle, the sexual drive and the physiological changes that take place during intercourse.

If the surgeon has to remove them totally – a practice that, with the advances in medical science, is becoming more and more rare – he will prescribe a substitute hormonal treatment immediately after the operation.

In this way, the patient will avoid all the inconveniences of menopause – hot flushes, insomnia, drying of the vagina and loss of libido – and her sex life will not be affected.

The operation is carried out under general or local anaesthetic. A horizontal incision is made in the stomach at the level of the pubis, so that the scar remains hidden even when wearing a bikini.

Just a reminder that the ovaries are two glands found either side of the uterus and measuring about three centimetres long and two centimetres thick. The right-hand ovary is often a little larger than the left-hand one.

FEMALE SURGICAL STERILIZATION

This operation makes fertilization impossible. The surgeon cuts the tubes and ligatures them, so preventing the spermatozoons from passing through to the egg.

The operation, which is carried out under general anaesthetic, is either done through laparotomy (abdominal incision) or laparoscopy (introduction under the navel of a little periscope which lights up the inside of the stomach and through which surgical instruments can be used).

In the first case, there will be a small scar around the pubic hairs. In the second case, there will be no visible trace of an operation. The length of hospitalisation is between two and ten days. And sexual intercourse can be resumed very quickly afterwards.

Surgical sterilization is final and anyone who undergoes it must give up all hope of future pregnancy. So any decision must take into consideration the irreversible consequences. Both medical and therapeutical advice are indispensable.

Only those motives based on reasons acknowledged by the doctor will be accepted – for example the risk of bringing into the world an abnormal child if one of the partners has a genetic problem, cancer or mental illness.

In no event can surgical sterilization be considered as a method of contraception. Even for a woman who cannot put up with any of the classic forms of contraception (be it the pill, the coil or the diaphragm), this should never be thought of as an option. There still remains the practice of coitus interruptus (the withdrawal of the penis before ejaculation) or the use of a condom.

HORMONAL SKIN PATCHES

Prescribed by the doctor in the case of hormone deficiency, these enable the medicine to pass through the skin, thus avoiding the risk of the products being absorbed by the digestive system. This method is also known as Hormone Replacement Therapy (HRT).

The principal application is in the treatment of menopause, whether natural or brought on by an ovariectomy (removal of the ovaries by surgery). In either case, the ovaries no longer produce the ovules necessary for reproduction and the secretion of sexual hormones (oestrogens and progesterone) is no longer assured. The consequences affect the psychological equilibrium as much as the physical and sexual health.

One notices a drop in sexual appetite, a drying of the vagina which can make intercourse painful, a deficiency in the bone density leading to the risk of osteoporosis, problems with sleeping, hot flushes and a general state of nervousness and worry. A hormone treatment is required: pills, capsules or patches.

This last form offers major advantages. For a start, since the medicine passes through the skin, it does not travel through the liver which would otherwise make the hormones inactive. The dose is weaker, so there is less chance of a rise in blood pressure or an increase in the blood's fat level.

Another advantage is the ease of use. The patch, which comes in a sealed sachet, is removed at the moment of application. It is placed on the hip or the shoulder, where it sticks to the skin and is resistant to all contact with water, even a shower or bath.

The treatment must be by doctor's prescription, which will indicate the number of patches to be used during the cycle.

Generally this is a long term treatment. There may be some side effects, but these are fairly rare. If they do occur, they will manifest themselves mostly in the form of itching and significant blotching. If there are any side effects at all it will be necessary to consult the doctor immediately.

THE COUPLE AND SEXUAL HEALTH

SEXUAL HYGIENE

The care one takes over bodily cleanliness, which is part of everyday life, must quite obviously be extended to cover the sexual organs – for one's own sake and that of one's partner.

However, one should also be aware that the fragile membranes that secrete a mucus which protects them against external attack must not be subjected to over-energetic treatment.

For the woman

The vulva – that is to say the outer and inner lips, the urinary meatus and the clitoris – is made of skin covered with a more or less abundant fleece. One should wash this gently with soap, sliding a finger between the folds.

As for the vagina, it is not recommended to clean the inside, either with soap or just water. In effect, the mucous membranes lining it secrete a 'flora' which protects it from any germs penetrating from the outside. So, save in the case of a recognized infection which needs medical treatment, there should be no internal washing of this organ – nor injections nor vaginal douches.

After making love and during the monthly periods, the same rules should be respected. Blood does not linger in the vagina. It is expelled by the menstrual flux and any residue absorbed by the mucous membrane. At all times the vagina remains naturally clean.

For the man

Daily washing of the penis, the bursae and the pubic hair is indispensable. And those not circumcised must uncover their glans and wash this too to prevent the formation, in the folds of the foreskin, of the whitish deposit known as smegma, which gives off an unpleasant smell.

TOBACCO AND SEXUALITY

The harmful effects of tobacco on the heart and the blood vessels have been scientifically demonstrated. For men, tobacco can also have a harmful repercussion on erections, which are provoked by the rush of blood into the hollow spongy body of the penis.

Nicotine causes the vessels and arteries that carry blood into the penis to contract and this in turn slows down the flow of blood. Moreover, nicotinism also reaches the nerve centres which, through a complex mechanism, transmit sexual excitement. The erection will then no longer have the same quality and may sometimes disappear, which can be a problem for heavy smokers and particularly those over fifty.

With women, the consequences of smoking on sexuality are equally heavy. Tobacco attacks one of the two female sexual hormones, the oestrogens, which are secreted by the ovaries. Linked with the other sexual hormone, the progesterone, oestrogens assure not only the continuity of the cycle and the right development of pregnancy, but also the burst of sexual desire and the physiological changes that help guarantee successful intercourse.

Moreover, it is also agreed that heavy smoking upsets the immune systems. Those who smoke a lot are particularly susceptible to localised infections brought on by bacteria and parasites, such as *Chlamydia, Trichomonas* and *Candida albicans*.

When an infection reaches the Fallopian tubes, these can be blocked and this results in terrible pains and sometimes even sterility. Because it is in these thready passages that the eggs produced by the ovaries travel. One single egg then lodges itself in a tube where the 'chosen' spermatozoon will go to meet it. With a blockage, no fertilization is possible.

We should also point out that menopause comes earlier for smokers than for non-smokers.

CHOLESTEROL AND SEXUAL HEALTH

Cholesterol is an organic substance present in all the cells of the human body, in the blood and in the bile, a bitter fluid secreted by the liver. Cholesterol is put into the body by food.

All men and women have some cholesterol, its role being notably that in the fabrication of the male and female sexual hormones. Blood contains 1.5-2.5 grammes of it. The excess is eliminated in the faeces and by the liver. A blood sample will enable one to know the level of cholesterol in the blood. Normally this must be below 2.5 grammes.

The laboratory report will indicate the levels of HDL, the 'good' cholesterol, and LDL and VLDL, the 'bad' cholesterols. It is the relationship between these levels which counts. The bad cholesterols risk being deposited on the walls of the blood vessels and forming patches of atheroma, which are responsible for filling the vessels and, as a result, cause cardiac troubles. In contrast, the good cholesterol is useful, even necessary, since it cleans the arteries.

An excess of bad cholesterols can lead to the formation of deposits in the very thin arteries that bring to the penis the blood that provokes the erection. If the blood flow in the penis is not working properly – or not at all – erection becomes difficult or even impossible. So one can understand the importance of the cholesterol in one's sex life.

High levels of cholesterol are not irremediable and can be treated with specific medicines and through a diet low in animal fats. This means avoiding meat, eggs, dairy produce and butter, for example. Vegetable oils and fish, on the other hand, are recommended. Alcohol is not advisable.

Recent research has shown that a high-fibre diet (oat flakes, for example) will help lower the cholesterol level.

THE EFFECT OF CERTAIN MEDICINES ON SEXUALITY

With men as with women, it can happen that a particular medical treatment can adversely affect one's sexuality: a drop in libido (the sexual appetite) or difficulties in performing the sexual act, for example.

Such is the case with anti-anxiety drugs, designed to reduce high blood pressure. Here the quality of erection is affected and the woman has delayed orgasms or fails to climax completely. Tranquilizers, too, especially when taken on a permanent basis, can produce the same upsetting effects.

Anti-cholesterol drugs, diuretics and hypnotics provoke problems with erection, while tricyclic anti-depressants are responsible for delayed ejaculation. With patients suffering from stomach disorders and treated with anti-acids, there is often a reduction in erection or even complete failure.

With some patients, the troubles appear from the very start of their treatment. With others, they can be delayed. As soon as one begins to experience sexual difficulties, it is important to speak to a doctor. Because the 'problem' medicines belong to 'families', he or she will be able to choose another product which will not have the same after-effects. In any event, one should not stop the treatment, but ask for another.

EXCESS ALCOHOL AND SEXUALITY

While taking the occasional alcoholic drink helps get rid of inhibitions, causes excitement and unbridles one's sensuality, the habitual consumption of excessive quantities does cause sexual problems.

For a man intoxicated by alcohol, we know that there is a drop in the sexual appetite and difficulties with erection and ejaculation. Everyone knows the aggressive – and sometimes even violent – behaviour of a man who has drunk too much. So one can understand the harmful effect alcoholism can have on one's marital relationship.

Not only is the sex life upset but normal communication becomes impossible. Moreover, the alcoholic often develops an irrational sense of jealousy. And when this happens with the woman, she equally sees her libido drop and experiences periods of both depression and aggression. She also feels demeaned by the disgust that her partner can show.

We are, of course, only talking here about true alcoholics, who have become totally dependent on large and regular quantities of alcohol.

It does happen that people who have, for example, been victims of a lack of affection or a psychological trauma look to drink to give them the strength to cope with their deep stress. To start with, they feel their condition improving... and therein lies the trap. By increasing the consumption of alcohol to relieve themselves of their problems, such men and women become on the contrary prisoners to drink.

When, with a couple, such a situation arises with one partner, the other must convince them of the need to see a doctor before the process of auto-intoxication causes even more serious damage to their overall health in general and their sexual health in particular.

INFECTIONS OF THE GENITAL ORGANS

Bacteria and parasites can develop in the genital organs, provoking unpleasant or painful irritations, and can then be transmitted to one's sexual partner.

When, for example, the *Candida albicans* – a fungal infection – migrates from the intestine, where it ordinarily lives, into the vagina, the woman will experience some abnormal white discharge and sharp feelings of burning on her vulva, in the vagina and sometimes even on her thighs and bottom. Fortunately a specific treatment of antibiotics, which must equally be taken by her partner, will destroy this mycosis in about a fortnight.

Chlamydia is a bacteria that provokes infections which reveal themselves in women through discharges and for the man through a slight running of the meatus of the penis. Although such symptoms are initially hardly noticeable, they mark the period of incubation (three weeks), after which a small lesion forms on the glans or the foreskin – and, in the woman's case, on the walls of the vagina.

Diagnosis comes from laboratory tests and the treatment for both partners involves the taking of antibiotics for three weeks.

Trichomona is a parasite that lodges in the vagina without revealing itself. It can 'wake up', at which time the woman experiences a profuse running of the vagina, feels some itching and is aware of the presence of miniscule sores on the vulva. A man infected by the parasite has a running of the urethra.

The couple must consult a doctor, since the problem risks causing various complications. A local oral treatment has proved effective.

Condylomes are small protuberances resembling warts, brought on by the presence of a virus, which form on the genito-anal mucous membrane – with men and women alike. Sexually transmittable, this viral infection demands serious treatment via a doctor depending on the state of the *condylomes* and the general condition of the patients.

All these infections, we must repeat, are sexually transmittable and both partners must be treated simultaneously.

Gonorrhoea

Commonly known as the 'clap', this sexually transmittable disease is caused by a bacteria – gonococcus. For the man, the first symptom is a strong burning feeling when urinating. This is caused by an irritation in the urethral canal, which runs past the prostate and along the length of the penis. Very quickly a clear seepage appears at the end of the penis, which then turns yellowish and purulent.

It is necessary to seek treatment as soon as the first signs appear. Antibiotics will be prescribed, the most efficient type being determined from laboratory tests.

Gonorrhoea, also known as blennorrhagia, is sexually transmittable and so there should be no sexual intercourse during the treatment and not until further analysis has confirmed that the patient is cured. The partner must be warned and submit herself to an examination to see whether she too has been infected.

With women, the signs of infection by gonococcus are inflammation of the vulva and the vagina and more or less profuse yellow discharges. They become evident between two and ten days after intercourse. Equally there can be a problem urinating.

Sometimes the symptoms are so slight that the woman does not feel any concern. Despite that, it is imperative that she sees a doctor and is treated in order to avoid any future complication such as infection of the neck of the uterus and the Fallopian tubes, which risks leading to sterility.

Genital herpes

Extremely contagious, the sexually transmitted disease is characterized by small erosions on the genital parts of the male (around the anus, the gland, the foreskin and the sheath of the penis) or those of the female (the inner lips, the entrance of the vagina, the anal region and the neck of the uterus).

The cause is a virus, which can remain dormant for a long time in the nerve glands found either side of the bottom part of the vertebral column and can be brought to life under the effect of over-tiredness, psychological stress or an infection.

First the victim experiences itching and local burning. Some hours later, a red blotch appears. This becomes covered with miniscule vesicles which open to release a clear fluid. These eruptions are very painful. Following this, a crust forms over the vesicles and eventually falls off. There is no scar. The attack, which lasts between five and ten days, is accompanied by intense fatigue and sometimes fever.

Because of the very contagious nature of genital herpes, it is imperative that the sufferer abstains from all sexual intercourse from the very first signs of the disease, warns his or her partner and sees a doctor.

Now there is an anti-herpetic gel which acts against the pain and the length of the attack of genital herpes. However, in nearly half the cases, there is a recurrence and herpes can even become chronic.

While this disease is not really serious, it is certainly uncomfortable for the victim, particularly as regards sexual activity. It should be noted, too, that for a woman who is pregnant herpes in the neck of the uterus can contaminate the baby in the course of childbirth, with a major risk of giving it meningitis or causing blindness. The obstetrician, who is the sole judge of the seriousness in each instance, will decide whether or not to perform a caesarean.

AIDS

This is the most formidable of sexually transmitted diseases since as yet one does not know how to cure it. The letters, incidentally, stand for Acquired Immunization Deficiency Syndrome.

Our body manufactures antibodies, which ensure protection against microbes and viruses. But this system of protection does not function in the case of the HIV virus, whicn is responsible for AIDS.

This virus can be transmitted through sperm, vaginal secretions, transfusion of contaminated blood and contaminated syringes. HIV can equally be present in saliva, tears, urine or faeces, although here its concentration is too weak to be dangerous.

The disease, which is diagnosed through a blood test, can attack heterosexuals as well as homosexuals, the groups most at risk being drug addicts and bisexuals, transfused haemophiliacs and homosexuals.

The presence of anti-HIV antibodies reveals seropositivity and their absence seronegativity. To be seropositive signifies that the subject has been in contact with the virus.

In order not to transmit the virus, it is imperative for the man to warn his partner, use condoms every time he has sexual intercourse and give up all oral sex. In the case of a woman, she must use an effective method of contraception, since the virus can be transmitted to a child. Mothers who are breast-feeding should stop immediately, since their milk could equally transmit the virus.

During the first stage of seropositivity, there are no symptoms whatsoever. The second stage is marked by a weakening of the immune defences. And it is at the third stage that AIDS develops, that is to say a total breakdown of the immune system. Following that come infections which, although not serious for an otherwise healthy person, can be fatal.

10

SOME QUESTIONS AND ANSWERS

*Talking with the sexologist:
a look at some of the topics that fascinate and frighten*

Is it perverse for a man to ask his partner to shave her pubis? And is it normal, for her part, to agree to such a wish?

This does not amount to perversion, but the search for novelty, a taste of something different which is common with a lot of men. Changing the outward appearance of your sexual organ can be a source of erotic excitement. As for the woman, it is up to her to decide whether she is prepared to do it or refuse to give in to her partner's wishes. But there is absolutely no problem here, except the inconvenience of having to continue to shave or pluck the hairs to keep the pubis clean-shaven.

Does a woman run the risk of getting pregnant if she has sexual intercourse during her periods?

The risk is small, but it does exist where intercourse takes place towards the end of a long period (about eight days). Advanced ovulation can then lead to fertilization.

Does the sexual urge die off with age?

The results of a survey carried out in the United States by the University of San Francisco on 202 people over the age of eighty revealed that 88 per cent of men and 71 per cent of women still felt the urge to be loved and have sexual intercourse, 67 per cent of men and 33 per cent of women still had intercourse and 72 per cent of men and 40 per cent of women still masturbated.

How do young girls who are still virgins bleed during their periods?

For those girls whose hymen (the membrane at the entrance of the vagina) is intact, blood has no difficulty in flowing since the hymen is pierced with a small hole which allows for this flow. It can happen – although it is rare – that this opening does not exist. Then the blood cannot flow and accumulates inside, leading to pains in the lower abdomen. In such a case, treatment must be sought. This involves making a slight incision in the hymen.

Does a woman who swallows her partner's sperm risk becoming pregnant?

No. Sperm that is swallowed passes through the digestive tube which is in no way linked with the female reproductive organs.

Does the fact of only having one testicle have any influence on one's sex life?

A man with only one testicle can have a completely normal sex life. This is not exceptional. Testicles form in the stomach of the foetus and move down progressively towards the line of the groin before leaving and taking their place in the scrotum. But it can happen that only one testicle completes the journey. It is possible, before puberty, to encourage this descent either by medical treatment or an operation. Even if this has not been done, the sexual function is not especially affected and the production of spermatozoons is sufficient to ensure fertilization of one's partner as often as the couple wish it.

What are wet dreams?

These are ejaculations which, for the most part, happen when one is asleep, during an erotic dream of which one does not have the least recall. In general they are accompanied by a real orgasm which often wakes the subject up to damp sheets. Nothing is more normal and no moral judgement should be passed on such spontaneous ejaculations.

Is it possible to test for a man's virginity?

Not at all. When a man makes love for the first time, there is absolutely no change in his anatomy – unlike a woman, who loses her hymen. Thus virginity remains totally symbolic for a man.

Can one have a prolonged erection without ejaculating?

This is quite a frequent phenomenon. An erection comes, for example, when one is watching an erotic or pornographic film or during a deeply amorous flirtation. This can cause in the lower abdomen, in the muscles of the perineum, an uncomfortable contracting and itchy feeling. Such discomfiture is not serious and will go away on its own in a few hours after the penis has relaxed. Some men find the need to relieve themselves by masturbating to bring on ejaculation.

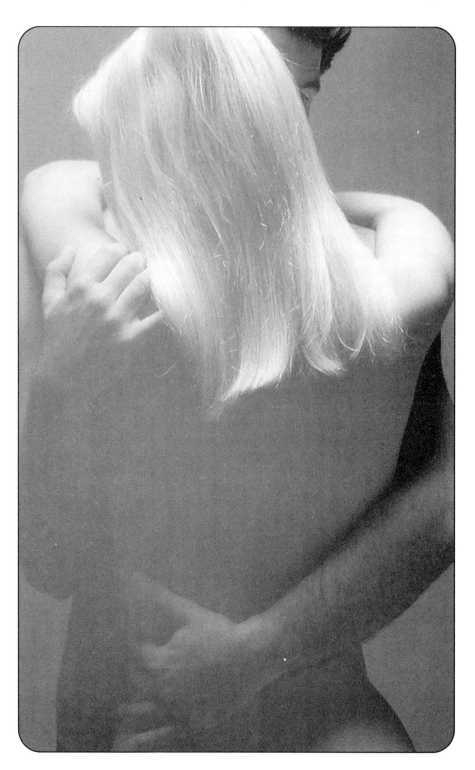

Up to what age does a man remain fertile?

Right up to the end of his life. However, after sixty the quantity of sperm released is less profuse and the spermatozoons become less fertile. They are, nevertheless, perfectly capable of fertilization.

Is love-making dangerous for heart patients?

According to a report from the Swiss Cardiological Foundation, 100 per cent of men and 75 per cent of women give up sexual intercourse after having a cardiac arrest. However a Japanese study in 1989, carried out on 5,500 cases of sudden death, showed that only thirty-four occured during sexual intercourse. In the normal course of events, doctors do not forbid heart patients from having sex. However, they do recommend a certain moderation in the frequency.

Does excess weight affect sexual behaviour?

It is necessary to clarify what one means by excess weight. One can talk about obesity when one is ten kilos (one stone six pounds) overweight. In this case, while one's sexual appetite is not generally affected, especially for a man the realisation may well be. To obtain and retain an erection becomes difficult, even among young people. In addition, obese people show a tendency to be lazy and apathetic. They are hardly daring when it comes to love. Psychologically they are often ashamed of their body and those areas of excessive fat and do not want to be seen undressed. This attitude is common, particularly among women. To conclude from this that all fat people are bad lovers would certainly be an exaggeration. Indeed, certain men and women, even thin ones, feel a particular attraction towards 'well-covered' people.

How long can one keep condoms?

You will often find a 'use by' date on condom packets. The period one can keep them for varies, according to the brand, from three to five years. They should be kept dry, cool and away from sunlight.

What causes erections at night and in the morning?

Scientific studies on male sexuality have shown that a man under sixty-five and in good health can have an erection every ninety minutes. An erection can occur during sleep or at the moment of waking up, with dreams or subconscious erotic thoughts.

Does slimming lead to a loss of sexual appetite?

It all depends on how one is slimming. If this involves a well-balanced diet, the loss of weight has no effect on one's sexuality.

On the other hand, if the diet includes the taking of certain medicines, then the sexual urge can diminish.

If, during childbirth, it is necessary to cut the vaginal mucous membrane, the muscles in the orifice of the vagina and the skin, does sexual intercourse become painful for the woman?

These surgical measures, which are designed to ease the passage of the baby's head, leave no other traces than some thin scars which later often become invisible. This mini-operation is called episiotomy. When the woman recommences sexual intercourse, the timing of which will be determined by the gynaecologist, she may feel some burning and gnawing pains which will disappear quite quickly. The real problem can be a psychological one. Just the fear of pain can lead her to avoid or refuse intercourse. In such cases, the woman should go and see her doctor, to check that the operation has not left any abnormal traces, and a psychotherapist to recover her enjoyment of sex.

Does the operation on the prostate lead to impotence?

The man becomes sterile but not impotent. He can still ejaculate, but the sperm is not projected towards the end of the penis but sent back towards the bladder. We call this physiological phenomenon backward ejaculation. His sex life and the possibility for orgasm are not affected.

Does the removal of the ovaries mark the end of a woman's sex life?

Absolutely not. Whether one or two ovaries are removed or just a part of this female sexual gland, the urge and pleasure are in no way affected. This operation, an ovariectomy, results in sterility, the end of periods and sometimes an increase in weight, which can be checked with the appropriate hormone treatment.

Can medicines have a noticeable effect on sexuality?

For men and women alike, some do have negative effects. These include the medicines prescribed for high blood pressure, anti-depressants, tranquilizers, diuretics and anti-cholesterol drugs, any of which can react on the sexual appetite and also the act of love-making: difficulties with erection for the man and delayed orgasm – or none at all – for the woman. In such circumstances one should consult the doctor with a view to changing the treatment.

Can a woman have sexual intercourse during her periods?

From a medical point of view, there is nothing to stop this. One should however take into account the risk of pregnancy, since the woman can be fertilized during these periods.

What is andropause?

This is a period between the ages of fifty and sixty when a man experiences a decline in his sexual activity and suffers different problems: indigestion, tiredness and depression. Not all men go through andropause – and in fact some doctors challenge its very existence. To avoid its effects, one should lead a healthy life, refrain from the excesses of alcohol and food, take plenty of exercise and especially maintain some sexual activity. A hormone treatment available on prescription is generally effective.

Is love-making tiring?

Absolutely not. The energy one exerts for this corresponds to that used up in the course of jogging a hundred metres. However, if love-making takes place several times during the day and the night, it can prove tiring – just as after any prolonged physical effort.

During sexual intercourse lasting three minutes:

* one's breathing rhythm increases to 40 breaths a minute during the excitement phase and reaches 60 breaths a minute during orgasm.
* one's heartbeats increase to 100-120 a minute during the excitement phase and reach 160-180 a minute during orgasm.

Is alcohol a stimulant for love?

In small amounts, alcohol can be a beneficial stimulant. It removes inhibitions and so allows one to display one's emotions more freely and have the courage to be more sensual in one's caressing. On the other hand, drunkenness is the enemy of love. A man can find he has difficulties with erection and tiredness can overtake one's efforts to succeed. It is worth pointing out that true alcoholics enjoy a very mediocre – and often a non-existent – sex life.

Can a pregnant woman have sexual intercourse?

Barring any medical advice to the contrary, a pregnant woman can continue to enjoy a normal sex life. Up to the third month, while her stomach is still flat, any of the positions can be practised. But from the fourth month, one must adopt only those where the man is positioned behind the woman and avoid too deep or violent penetration. The foetus runs absolutely no risk during coitus – even up to the end of the pregnancy. But one must however discuss the situation with one's gynaecologist on each prenatal visit.

Do aphrodisiac foods really exist?

Certain foods rich in vitamins and mineral salts are beneficial to the whole body, helping to provide a general tonic which consequently boosts one's sexual energy as well. Such, among other things, is the case with celery, chick peas, truffles, fish eggs and numerous spices – cinnamon, coriander, ginger, mint, chilli and saffron – with which it is easy to season dishes and which can be used to make herbal teas, elixirs and envigorating wines.

Is vasectomy irreversible?

This operation, which consists in sectioning the deferent ducts which carry the spermatozoons from the testicles to the prostate, where they mix together with the prostatic fluid to form sperm, is a radical form of surgical contraception. It makes the man sterile for good. However, those who have had the operation continue to enjoy a normal sex life, because vasectomy affects neither the quality of erection nor the pleasure of orgasm. Ejaculation still occurs, but the fluid no longer contains any sperm.

How long after childbirth can a woman make love again?

From the moment when there is no more loss of blood following the delivery, that is to say two or three weeks after childbirth. One will have to add several more weeks if there has been an episiotomy (incision of the vulva) to enable the passage of the baby's head. It is then necessary to wait until the scar has healed completely.

Must people playing sport abstain from sexual intercourse before a competition?

This is an old-fashioned theory which was nurtured over the centuries though ancient custom whereby certain tribes indulged in all kinds of orgies to honour their gods before going into combat. These tired warriors lost plenty of battles. But there is a world of difference between orgies and normal love-making. In fact, recent scientific studies have shown that the sexual act calms the body and the mind. It is the best anti-stress recipe for a champion. Figures speak for themselves. During a coitus of three minutes, the breathing rhythm mounts to 60 breaths a minute during orgasm and, at the same time, heartbeats are 160-180 a minute. But these return to normal within about three minutes. Not only does the sportsman not suffer any adverse effects, but during sexual intercourse hormone secretions of testosterone, in particular, are produced. Not only is this the hormone of desire, but also of combativeness. One now knows that sportsmen do not have to go on a sexual fast. The length of time one should allow between making love and competing in an event varies from person to person – from just a few minutes to up to six hours.

Does the use of tobacco affect one's sexual capability?

With men, nicotine has an adverse effect on erection, provoking a contraction of the vessels that carry blood into the cavernous body of the penis and thus ensure its volume and rigidity. With women, nicotine brings equally adverse effects in provoking a slowing-down of the blood-flow in the genital organs, which results in creating difficulties with vaginal lubrication. And we know that the drying of the vagina makes intercourse difficult and sometimes even painful.

What is the difference between leucorrhoea and vaginal lubrication?

Vaginal lubrication is a transudation – or, more simply, sweating – of the vagina which happens at the moment when a woman is sexually excited. This sweating is accompanied by secretions of the Bartholin glands, located either side of the vaginal opening. Leucorrhoea has nothing at all to do with the sexual urge. Its origin is an infection, brought on by the presence of a germ, mycosis or trichomonas. In the majority of cases it will disappear following gynaecological treatment.

Is it true that, at the age of puberty, boys' breasts can develop in the same way as girls'?

Male puberty does sometimes bring this type of physical change, due to the awakening of the hormones, which are produced at this time. There is, however, no cause for alarm since these indications disappear of their own accord after a few months.

Is the question of contraception down to the woman?

In any well-balanced relationship, this is a subject that must be dealt with in perfect calmness. In many cases, women have been using contraceptives since their adolescence. But a lot of gynaecologists and sexologists are agreed that some women feel themselves slaves to contraception and want, at least temporarily, to free themselves from it. Here it is essential that they can talk about it with their partner and suggest that he takes on part of the responsibility by using a condom. The withdrawal method is not recommended, since it demands perfect control on the man's behalf and, even still, a few spermatozoons can be released before ejaculation. Equally, it is frustrating for both partners.

Can one put a coil on a retroverted uterus?

Yes, if it is a simple retroversion, that is to say if the uterus is facing forwards or backwards, which is the case with about 20 per cent of women. A mobile muscle, the uterus can moreover change position when it is pushed by neighbouring organs – the bladder, for example. But you cannot put a coil on a retroverted uterus that has lost its mobility and is attached to adjoining organs. This is rare and generally due to a former and treated problem – such as peritonitis, for example.

Is there a contraceptive pill for men?
Actually not. A male contraceptive pill is very difficult to create since there is not in a man's life a comparable cycle to that of a woman – or ovulation, which served as the basis on which the pill was created for women. Research was conducted by the World Health Organisation, but has been abandoned due to the lack of any encouraging results.

What is anal love?
This sexual practice, which is called sodomy, involves the intromission of the penis into the anus. An act both homosexual and heterosexual, sodomy is not without risk since the anus, restricted by a powerful sphincter, does not offer the same chances of distension as the vagina. Penetration can be painful and cause lacerations and, after a time, stretching of the anus. However, because the anus is a richly innervated area, some do take pleasure in this practice.

INDEX

Accomplice position 138
AIDS 289-90
Alcohol 266, 286-7, 296
Amazon position 153
Amenorrhea 276-7
Anal sex 299
Anaphrodisia 238-41
Androgens 267
Andropause 256-7, 296
Angelica infusions 260
Anorgasmia 238, 241
Aphrodisiacs 261-2, 263-6, 297
Auto-eroticism 30-2, 62, 225, 269
  see also Fantasies

Bartholin glands 20, 65, 275
Beauty, complexes about 36-7
Big Shiver position 151
Biofeedback, premature ejaculation 227
Birth control 243-51
  coil 244-5, 249-50, 298-9
  coitus interruptus (withdrawal method) 31, 224, 225, 247-8, 251
  condoms 246-7, 289-90, 294
  diaphragm 245-6, 250
  making love for first time 46
  pill 243-4, 248-9, 299
  responsibility for 298
  spermicides 245, 246, 250-1
  sterilization 270-1, 282, 297
  temperature method 247, 251
Blennorrhagia 288
Boat position 144
Body awareness 16-30
  see also Genital organs; Health matters
Body complexes 36-7
Body hair 17-18, 20, 28, 284, 291
Body language 32-4
Breasts 16, 66, 67, 76
  men 28-9, 69, 298
Breathing, during lovemaking 66, 69, 296
Bride (penis) 269
Buggery 299
Bull position 119

Butterfly position 136

Calcium 261, 262, 281
Candida albicans 287
Captive position 102
Cardiac arrest, sex after 294
Caressing 51, 53, 55
Caressing Love position 183
Cervix (collar of uterus) 21, 22, 74, 75
Childbirth 20, 77-8, 278, 295, 297
Chlamydia 287
Cholesterol 285-6
Cigarette smoking 284-5, 298
Circumcision 27, 269
Clap, the 288
Clitoris 18, 64, 259
Coaxer position 114
Coil, the 244-5, 249-50, 298-9
Coitus interruptus (withdrawal method) 31, 224, 225, 247-8, 251
Condoms 246-7, 289-90, 294
Condylomas 288
Contraception *see* Birth control
Conversation position 195
Copper 261, 263
Cunnilingus 58-9, 60-1, 239

Deferent ducts 29, 68, 271
Desire *see* Libido
Diaphragm 245-6, 250
Diet *see* Food
Divorce 210
Dominator position 100
Double Cavalcade position 131
Double Game position 146
Dysmenorrhea 277-8
Dyspareunia 237

Ejaculation 46, 53-4, 62, 68-9, 267
  backward 295
  coitus interruptus (withdrawal method) 31, 224, 225, 247-8, 251
  erection without 292
  feminine 23, 63
  kissing and 40
  premature 223-8, 248, 269

Ejaculation *(continued)*
  prostate gland 29, 270
  wet dreams 292
Endometriosis 274, 280-1
Episiotomy 77, 278, 295
Erections 25, 27, 228-9, 294
  from foreplay to orgasm 67-8
  making love for first time 46, 47
  obesity 294
  problems with 228-35, 261, 263, 269, 284, 285, 298
  size 219, 220
  without ejaculation 292
Erogenous zones 16, 19, 23-4, 29-30
Exchange position 109
Exhibitionism 92-5

Face-to-Face position 137
Fallopian tubes 21, 272, 274-5, 285
Fantasies 31, 81-8
Fellatio 58-60, 61-2, 292
Femininity, body awareness 16-25
Fetishism 88-90
Fibromas 271, 272, 278-9
Fidelity 205-6, 207-14
Fireworks position 162
Flirtation 37-9
Food
  aphrodisiacs and tonics 261-3, 297
  cholesterol 285-6
  osteoporosis prevention 281
  romantic recipes 263-6
  slimming diets 294-5
Foreplay 44, 46, 51-6, 56-8, 239
  see also Erogenous zones; Kissing
Foreskin 27, 68, 269, 284
Frigidity 238-41

G spot 22-3
Games 215-16
Gate of Paradise position 124
Gazelle position 178
Geisha position 168
Genital herpes 288-9
Genital organs
  men 25-30, 67-70, 219-23, 228-9, 256-8, 292
  women 16-25, 65-7, 76-7, 253-6, 258-9
  see also Health matters
Glans 25, 27, 68, 284
Gonorrhea 288
Greyhound position 175, 222
Gynaecological examination 271-2

Hair 17-18, 20, 28, 284, 291

Health matters
  cardiac arrest 294
  cholesterol 285-6
  effects of medicines 286, 295
  endometriosis 274, 280-1
  episiotomy 278, 295
  excess alcohol 286-7
  excess weight 294-5
  fibromas 271, 272, 278-9
  gynaecological examination 271-2
  hormone replacement 283
  hygiene 276, 284
  hysterography 274-5
  infections 276, 285, 287-90, 298
  laparoscopy 272, 274
  menstrual problems 276-8
  osteoporosis 281
  ovarian cysts 279-80
  ovariectomy 281-2, 295
  phimosis 27, 269
  prostate gland 269-70, 295
  sex hormones 267, 275-6
  slimming 294-5
  smoking 284-5, 298
  sperm 268-9
  surgical sterilization 282
  tonics 260-3
  ultrasound scan 272
  vaginal drying 276
  vasectomy 270-1, 297
  see also Pregnancy; Sexual problems
Heart disease, sex and 294
Heart rate, during lovemaking 66, 69-70, 296
Herbal tonics 260-1
Herpes, genital 288-9
HIV infection 289-90
Hop position 166
Hormones *see* Sex glands and hormones
Hug position 104
Hygiene 35-6, 276, 283-4
Hymen 20-1, 44, 46, 47, 291-2
Hypnosis, premature ejaculation 227
Hysterectomy 279
Hysterography 274-5

Impotence 228-35, 261, 263
Infections 276, 285, 287-90, 298
Inferiority complexes 36-7
Infidelity 205-6, 207-14
Infusions 260-1
Intercourse *see* Lovemaking
Interweaving position 112
Iron supplements 263

Jealousy 203-6

Kissing 39-43, 53

Laparoscopy 272, 274
Lazy Love position 193
Letters 13-15
Leucorrhea 298
Libido
  age factors 231, 256-7, 258,
    259, 260-3, 291, 296
  alcohol 286
  andropause 256-7, 296
  aphrodisiacs 261-2, 263-6, 297
  differences in 201, 207-8
  during pregnancy 75
  effects of medicines 286, 295
  fantasies for 82
  following childbirth 77-8
  frequency of intercourse 73-4
  frigidity 238-41
  hormonal skin patches 283
  infidelity 207-8
  love and 11-12
  menopause 258, 283
  premenstrual syndrome 235, 236
  romantic meals 263-6
  sexual weariness 214-17
  slimming and 294-5
  tobacco smoking 284-5
  tonics 260-3, 297
Long Distance position 157
Love
  desire and 11-12
  duration 12-13
  frequency of intercourse 72-4
Love letters 13-15
Love Trap position 120
Lovemaking
  for first time 44, 46-9
  frequency 72-4
  pain during 44, 46, 220-1, 237,
    269, 274
  positions 97-196, 216, 221-2
  seduction aids 34-5, 263-6
  see also Sexual problems
Loving Hold position 165
Lubrication, vaginal 20, 22, 46, 65,
  67, 76, 259, 276, 298

Magnesium 261, 262, 263
Massage 56-8
Master position 121
Masturbation 30-2, 62, 225, 269
  see also Fantasies
Meals, recipes 263-6

Medical problems *see* Health matters
Medicines, side effects 286, 295
Menstrual cycle 275
  amenorrhea 276-7
  dysmenorrhea 277-8
  endometriosis 280
  fertilization 268, 275, 291
  hormones 21
  hygiene 284
  hymen 291-2
  intercourse 291, 295-6
  iron supplements 263
  menopause 253-6, 258-9, 276,
    281, 283, 285
  premenstrual syndrome 235-6
Mineral salts 261-2, 262-3, 281
Missionary position 98, 216, 221
Mistress position 160
Mount of Venus (pubis) 17-18, 20, 291
Myomectomy 279

Nipples 16, 28-9, 66, 69, 76

Obesity 294-5
Odour, power of 35-6
Oestrogens 21-2, 77, 275
  menopause 254
  oral contraceptives 243-4
  osteoporosis and 281
  tobacco smoking 284-5
  vaginal dryness 276
Offering position 186
Onanism 31
Open Flower position 154
Opening position 194
Oral contraception 243-4, 248-9, 299
Oral sex 58-62, 239, 289, 292
Orgasm 62-71, 296
  female 47, 54, 63-7
    after childbirth 77
    after menopause 259
    clitoral 18, 64
    G spot 23
    in pregnancy 75, 76-7
    problems of 237-41
    vaginal 23, 64
  male 46, 53-4, 62-3, 64-5,
    67-70, 292
  simultaneous 64-5
Osteoporosis 281
Ovaries 21, 77, 275
  egg production 268
  gynaecological examination 272
  at menopause 254
  osteoporosis 281
  ovarian cysts 279-80
  ovariectomy 281-2, 295

Papaverine therapy 234–5
Paraphimosis 269
Passing Hand position 190
Penetration
  erection problems 229, 230
  kissing a symbol of 41
  lubrication 20, 22, 46, 65
  making love for first time 44, 46, 47
  pain on
    men 27, 269
    women 220–1, 237
  size of penis 220–2
Penis 25, 27, 228–9
  health matters 27, 269
  hygiene 284
  size 219–23
  see also Erections
Perfume 35, 36
Perineum 28, 222
Periods *see* Menstrual cycle
Personal hygiene 35–6, 276, 283–4
Pheromones 35–6
Phimosis 27, 269
Phosphorus 262, 263
Pill, the 243–4, 248–9, 299
Pivot position 129
Plant tonics 260–2
Plastic surgery, breasts 16
Positions, lovemaking 97–196, 216, 221–2
Potassium 261, 262
Pregnancy
  childbirth 20, 77–8, 278, 295, 297
  fertilization 268, 275, 291
  gynaecological examination 271
  lovemaking during 74–7, 296
  making love for first time 46
  oral sex and 292
  prevention of *see* Birth control
  ultrasound scan 272
  uterus during 21, 22
Premature ejaculation 223–8, 248, 269
Premenstrual syndrome 235–6
Prisoner position 185
Progesterone 21–2, 275
  the coil and 244, 245
  menopause 254
  oral contraceptives 243–4
  osteoporosis and 281
  tobacco smoking 284–5
Prostaglandin E1 therapy 227
Prostate gland 29, 68, 269–70, 295
Pubic hair 17–18, 20, 28, 284, 291
Pubis (Mount of Venus) 17–18, 20, 291

Quiet Love position 176

Relationships
  duration 12–13
  flirting 37–9
  inferiority complexes 36–7
  initiation 32–4
  love and desire 11–12
  love letters 13–15
  problems in 197–217
  seduction aids 34–5, 263–6
Rider position 111
Romantic meals 263–6
Royal jelly 262

Scents, power of 35, 36
Scissors position 189
Scrotum 28, 68–9
Seduction
  aids to 34–5, 263–6
  body language 32–4
  complexes and 37
See-Saw position 134
Selenium 262–3
Self-confidence 36–7
Self-examination 16–30
Seminal vesicles 29, 68
Sensual Ride position 171
Sex games 215–16
Sex glands and hormones
  men 28, 29, 256–7, 267
  tonics 262, 263
  women 21–2, 77, 275–6
    the coil 244, 245
    hormonal skin patches 283
    menopause 254, 259, 281
    oral contraceptives 243–4
    osteoporosis 281
    ovarian cysts 279, 279–80
    ovariectomy 281–2, 295
    tobacco smoking 284–5
    vaginal dryness 276
Sex therapy 231–2
Sexual desire *see* Libido
Sexual intercourse *see* Lovemaking
Sexual organs *see* Genital organs
Sexual problems 197–217
  alcohol 286–7
  boredom and weariness 214–17
  cholesterol as cause of 285–6
  communication 197–203
  due to medicines 286, 295
  dyspareunia 237
  erections and impotence 228–35, 261, 263, 269, 284, 285, 298
  infidelity 205–6, 207–14

Sexual problems *(continued)*
  jealousy 203-6
  premature ejaculation 223-8, 269
  premenstrual syndrome 235-6
  tobacco smoking 284-5, 298
  vaginismus 237-8
  see also Health matters; Libido
Sharing position 148
Simultaneous orgasm 64-5
Skene glands 20, 275
Smegma 269, 284
Smell, power of 35-6
Smoking, effects of 284-5, 298
Sodomy 299
Soft Surrender position 140
Soixante-neuf (69) 60
Speculum 271
Sperm and spermatozoa 268-9
  fertility 256-7, 294
  fertilization 268, 275
  at orgasm 68, 268
  production of 29, 267, 268-9
  uterus and 21
  see also Birth control
Spermicides 245, 246, 250-1
Splits position 173
Sport 297-8
Sterilization 270-1, 282, 297
Submissive position 133
Sweat glands 20

Taste, sense of 40
Temperature method, birth
  control 247, 251
Testicles 28, 29, 68-9, 267, 292
Testosterone 267, 297
Thrush (*Candida*) 287
Tobacco smoking 284-5, 298
Tonics 260-3, 297
Trichomonas 287, 298
Tropical position 126

Ultrasound examination 272
Urethra 18, 25, 29, 68, 269
Uterus 21, 22
  during orgasm 66, 75, 76-7
  endometriosis 274, 280-1

fibromas 271, 272, 278-9
gynaecological examination 271
hysterectomy 279
hysterography 274-5
in pregnancy 75, 76-7
retroverted 271, 298-9

Vagina 18, 20-1, 22
  after menopause 259
  during lovemaking 65-6, 67, 76-7
  exercises for 222
  gynaecological examination 271
  hygiene 284
  lubrication 20, 22, 46, 65, 67,
    76, 259, 276, 298
  making love for first time 44,
    46, 47
  in pregnancy 76-7
  problems of orgasm 237-8
  vaginal orgasm 23, 64
Vaginismus 237-8
Vas deferens (deferent ducts) 29,
  68, 271
Vasectomy 270-1, 297
Venereal diseases 287-9
Virginity
  the hymen 20-1, 44, 46, 47, 291-2
  making love for first time 44, 46-9
  male 44, 292
  symbolic value 38, 49
Virility 25-30, 220-1
Vitamins, as tonics 261, 262
Voluptuous position 107
Voyeurism 90-2
Vulva 18, 77, 278, 284, 295

Watching position 180
Waves of the Sea position 159
Wet dreams 292
Whirlpool position 143
Willing Greyhound position 175, 222
Wines, for romantic meals 266
Withdrawal method (coitus
  interruptus) 31, 224, 225, 247-8, 251
Wrestler position 116

Young She-Goat position 122